Through the Fire
A Caregiver's Journal

See, I have refined you, though not as silver;
I have tested you in the furnace of affliction
-Isaiah 48:10

Thankful for His care

Donna Hutcherson

Book One
For Those Who Care
- A Caregiver Series

Copyright © 2022 by Donna Hutcherson

All rights reserved, including the right to reproduce this book or portions thereof in any form whatsoever or by any means. No part of this book may be reproduced, stored in a retrieval system, or transmitted by any means without the written permission of the Author, except as provided by United States of America copyright law.

First Paperback edition May, 2022

Manufactured in the United States of America

Scriptures referred to in this book are taken from the most up-to-date versions of the Holy Bible published by Zondervan Publishing House and provided online by Biblegateway.com.

Cover artwork by Cyndi Steen
Author picture by Tim Kern of TK Photography

Imprint: Donna Hutcherson
Amarillo, TX

PAPERBACK ISBN: 979-8-9862304-0-5
EBOOK ISBN: 979-8-9862304-1-2
AUDIO ISBN: 979-8-9862304-2-9

To Christy and David

Flesh of my flesh. My joy. Aaron and Hur as the battle raged.
Together we have been forged *in the fire of affliction* and come out
changed, refined, better able to face life.
With love and commitment forever…
To God be the glory…

Table of Contents

	Foreword	i
	Preface	iii
	My Family	vi
1	October 3, 2014	1
2	The First Month	4
3	NeuroRehab	50
4	Preparing for Home	84
5	Home Sweet Home	90
6	Six Months and Counting	103
7	Marking One Year	127
8	Stroked Again - Reset the Rehab	132
9	Shared Lives	147
10	Two Years of Changed Lives	168
11	A New Home	174
12	Hard Times	181
13	How Quickly Things Change	196
14	Homebound	205
15	Changing Addresses	224
	Epilogue	230
	Afterword	235
	Appendix 1	236
	Appendix 2	239
	Bibliography	241
	About the Author	242

Foreword

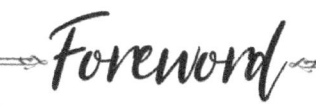

Stroke is a thief; and since there are few things more gratifying than to see tables turned and books balanced on a thief, I was happy to be included in this project. At first, I felt that a prominent Florida Gator football player or one of the extraordinarily capable specialists that worked with Dale would be a far better choice to write here, but I quickly saw Donna's wisdom: sadly, for all the great upheavals that it can cause, stroke is an everyday sort of thing. So, someone who has, for a time, simply walked through the day-to-day of a stroke's consequences in the lives of dear friends makes sense - to introduce this Journal and its invaluable perspective.

To be candid, I am thankful that I did not have to "live it" absolutely every day of the almost four years that this Journal recounts. That was Donna's experience, and Dale's. I was "involved" and "supportive," even "present" and "caring," from the first just-after-midnight calls and texts right to the very end. But that simply doesn't cut it. No one can understand what it is to have such a devastation make itself at home in the very heart of one's life. YET, that is this Journal's strength and triumph. It makes the impossible to experience accessible; and, for many, it will provide, reveal, a lifeline that will substantially enhance the lives of anyone and everyone touched by stroke whether patients and caregivers, or families and friends.

And not just stroke! That's the wonder and the promise of the whole endeavor. It is for ANY brain-altering disorder or traumatic injury or dementia (of which there are so many on the increase); for ANY debilitation that alters personality or perspective in a life-changing way; for ANY of the chronic diseases that DEMAND of the caregiver and the cared-for. To be sure, this Journal is grounded in the concerns and challenges, the experiences engendered by cerebrovascular accidents; and it will be a tremendous resource for those facing that particular assault, but its REACH is far more extensive. It ably demonstrates that ANY life-change born of disabling loss is not just an end, but truly a beginning.

It was one of the great joys of my life to see a man, who, by any standard of measure (for all that he had lost and endured) should have been crushed, defeated, and depressed, DANCING FOR JOY with his grandsons, HAPPY and FULFILLED, a mere handful of days before he began to experience the falls from which, ultimately, he would never rise. In this life.

THIS is his and his caregiver's story, told in all of its very human glory, highly personal, often urgent, sometimes unpolished, a Journal filled with practicalities and realities, of both sorrow and humor. Every brain, every injury, every sufferer (patient AND caregiver), every shared life, is unique. But this Caregiver's Journal, which I trust will help you not merely to survive but to thrive as you discover your own God-led way of caring for the changed person that you love, can be YOUR story of victory against all odds too. Just read it. You will find yourself in it.

- Sam Steen, MA
Brain Injury and Behavioral Specialist

Preface

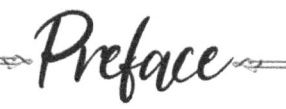

September 30, 2014

At age sixty-three, I retired, having spent my life's work in both education and business. My husband, Dale, had retired June 2012 from teaching and coaching after thirty-eight years. In the months approaching my retirement, our daughter, Christy, had asked several times what my plans were for "after." At that time, my answer was simple. I had many interests but no specific plans; Dale and I had trusted God for decades to unfold the plans He had for us and I was certain that would continue.

Three Days Later… October 3, 2014

While Dale and I were traveling out of town to join my sister and brother-in-law for a North Carolina vacation, Dale suffered a massive stroke (later, MRI revealed there were actually two strokes). This was six days short of his 64th birthday.

In a heartbeat, I now had a new full-time job… as Dale's caregiver.

"A man's heart plans his way, but the Lord directs his steps."
Proverbs 16:9

After four years of caring for Dale, I firmly believe that those individuals in a 24/7 primary caregiving role need all the help they can get in order to maintain their own personal well-being as well as that of the person for whom they are caring.

From the start of this caregiving journey, I *needed* God's help; the Truth is we all need God's help. And I trust that He, Who knows *everything* about every situation in which I find myself, also knows how to help me best handle whatever I'm facing. The key to gaining this knowledge that caregivers need to *survive* is to have a relationship with our Good, Kind, Loving, Heavenly Father. His Word tells us that He cares (I Peter 5:9). His Word tells us what we need to do to have Him live within us and guide us by His Holy Spirit (John 14, esp. v.15-17, 23). And His Word tells us how to hear His voice (John 10:3-4,11; Isaiah 30:21).

Relying on this relationship with our Heavenly Father is <u>the single most important thing one can do</u> as a caregiver; it's not simply <u>*my*</u> idea of how one should carry out responsibilities.

<u>*My*</u> *opinion means nothing*; **God's Truth is Life**.

As my life experience simply tells of His Love and Wisdom, it too will bring life. The only way in which we humans can fully function in a *healthy* manner under the external stressors that a caregiver faces daily is by Holy Spirit's guidance. And He graciously, lovingly shows us the way step by step as we *s-l-o-w* down enough to listen for the answers. Yes, answers will be there at the right time, maybe not as fast as we'd like, and sometimes not even <u>the answers we'd like</u>, but definitely at the right time as we need, one-step-at-a-time.

Most of the writings in this book are highly personal, originally told in real time, evolving from ACTUAL entries in both my public and my private journals and were initially penned to inform our family and friends of the journey in which both Dale and I were engaged. So you as a reader will be exposed to my heart and our lifestyle; for that I cannot apologize as you step into my life. Additionally, as typically happens when I write, putting pen to paper became a wellspring of clarity for me, often bringing into focus that intuitive aspect that gave light to our next step, assisting me in managing the unmanageable and ultimately revealing insights about HOW to continue living successfully and with joy.

At times, I hesitated to tell certain experiences in this journal; it can be pretty raw. And then, unexpectedly, I'd receive a note that our journey had inspired someone to be strong in spirit and faith. After telling God, *"I'm tired of being an inspiration,"* I'd repent of my selfishness, and over and over again yield to His plan to use me in whatever way serves Him and others best. He is the Potter; I am the clay. This lump of clay certainly doesn't claim to know what the Potter is making *or* His purpose; I choose to yield and let Him make me what He wills for His purposes, now and throughout eternity.

Knowing that I personally have gained SO MUCH COURAGE AND INSIGHT from the writings of others who've gone through life's trials before or alongside of me, how can I not openly share my life that others may be encouraged as well?

My prayer is that you will be blessed as you read, encouraged as you consider, and strengthened as you walk out your caregiving days.

Always thankful,

Donna Hutcherson

*always giving thanks to
God the Father for
everything, in the name of
our Lord Jesus Christ.
Ephesians 5:20 NIV*

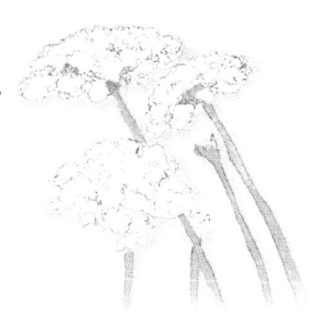

My Family

In this journal, my family is foremost, and you'll see their names throughout. Our lives are deeply intertwined. It is my privilege to introduce them to you.

Dale, my husband of forty-seven years (together since were eighteen), taught high school science and coached football, volleyball, and nearly every sport for thirty-eight years. We raised our family in Englewood, FL, where we finally retired. A brilliant man who loved young people, he lived to teach *everyone anything* he could *anytime*. His greatest post-stroke frustration was to no longer easily impart his life experience to help others. His greatest post-stroke sadness was to no longer be able to readily teach and coach his grandchildren. *But he never quit trying...*

Christy, beloved firstborn, follower of Christ, proud aunt to her three nephews, lives 1½ hours south of me, teaches high school science, and coaches several sports just like her dad (and travels wherever she can just like me). She is generous in giving, loyal in friendships, fierce in what she believes, steadfast and tenderhearted, and is always ready to help others. I value her insights, wisdom, travel expertise and friendship.

David, faithful son, God-follower, devoted husband, father and brother, lives ten minutes away from me, works in finance for a family-owned marine company, and captains a fishing charter. He understood his father better than anyone and had Dale's implicit trust. I value his male perspective, financial insights, emotional stability, steadfast loyalty, and prowess on the water.

Stephanie, David's wife of twenty-one years, is thankfully another daughter to me, lover of God, master homemaker, family glue, talented, creative, and a gift to our family. I value her courage and tenacity and the way she makes my son happy.

Joshua, **Matthew**, and **Caleb** are the precious sons of David and Stephanie and a constant source of joy to their grandparents (on both sides). Their dedication, honest feedback, and availability to us provided a constant source of life and laughter throughout our homebound days. It has been our joy and pleasure to live close enough to be involved as they grow into fine, engaging young men.

Lin, our daughter from another mother who joined our family as a high school senior, is now a homeschooling mom and life organizer, God-follower, overcomer, essential oils enthusiast, and a developing creative expressive arts facilitator.

Mike, Lin's husband of twenty-five years, is a Godly man with a brilliant mind, a sound thinker, coffee aficionado, and a software programmer who swept Lin away from Florida to a cooler climate.

Rebekah, **Hadassah**, and **Isaac**, Lin and Mike's three children, are precious to Dale and me, and yet, as they lived clear across the country, our personal visits over the years were few. After Dale's stroke when we could no longer travel that distance, this wonderful family created unique ways to support us, not the least of which were humor, research, and prayer. FaceTime helped us keep in touch and gave them a sense of Dale's abilities as well as impairments.

Our siblings and their spouses have shared life together with us over decades, through highs and lows and everything in between. Our family is blessed with deep relationships and great love: **Carol** and husband **Dale**; **Nancy** and husband **Ken**; **Rick** and wife **Melodie**; **Patti** and husband **Bill**; Dale's sister **Kim** and husband **Kevin** and a dozen nieces and nephews plus their spouses and children.

The brain is always changing, which continually brings hope.

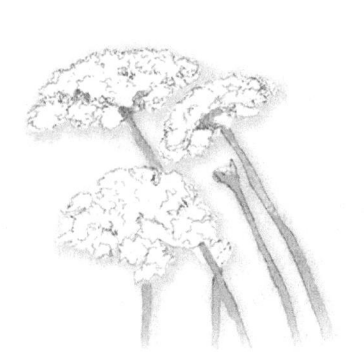

Chapter One

OCTOBER 3, 2014

10/3/14 - Pre-Stroke Afternoon

Driving to Amelia Island on our way to meet Nancy and Ken for vacation celebrating my retirement on September 30th, Dale drove as far as Gainesville and we changed drivers. By the time we got to Waldo twenty minutes later, he was complaining of a BAD headache and had taken 800 mg Ibuprofen™ which didn't touch the headache. He asked for and took the 1½ tablets of his muscle relaxer that I normally carry with me for him. Thirty minutes later, he was still hurting badly. I offered a couple of times to go to a hospital, but he declined, changing positions, and stretching out to adjust circulation, then sitting up holding his head. We were in a downpour, but I finally stopped to pull under a gas station overhang to consider what to do. Again, he said no to the hospital and asked for one more muscle relaxer from his suitcase in hopes of knocking this out. He fell asleep…then, another thirty minutes later, we were checking in at the Florida House in Amelia Island. He woke up on his own when we stopped and was groggy but went to the room to lie down, taking off his jewelry, shoes, glasses as normal, and putting his phone on the nightstand before stretching out. I told him I'd walk around and get some dinner and was gone about an hour. He was still asleep when I returned, so I prepared everything to leave early in the morning, then journaled, with lights out by 8:30 p.m. He woke up as I was settling down, talked with me a bit, then went back to sleep.

My Journal Entry That Night - Pre-Stroke

8:00 p.m. Amelia Island - First day of retirement trip! After an intense few days of preparation, I am SO grateful for time to relax.

Dale has been challenged for the past ten or so days—new glasses, packing, changes with memory, using remote, audio directions, and his concern about that. Talking some about it, but not much, but it's evident to me so I've been prayerful. It's definitely a huge adjustment for us both.

I'm recognizing more and yielding to patience and listening to precious Holy Spirit; His timing, not mine. God knows exactly where we are with all this, and He is faithful to lead.

Blessings continue to abound; I am so grateful for those who are helping with retirement transition:
- pastor's encouragement/prophecy that doors will open before us, that we have given and now it's time to receive
- David's advice to see our financial adviser and the ensuing gracious and wise advice
- dear friends we saw for insurance help – a joy to reconnect!
- Dale's desire to go to San Diego for ISM and my manager's willingness to offer that option
- a former student for our accountant - an unexpected gift
- piano teacher for the boys; my enjoyment of working with them on piano
- boys' love of chess; Dale's gift of good chess sets - done!
- recommendation of *Searching for Bobby Fischer* movie

Stroke!

Florida House is the oldest hotel in Florida and has little insulation; so, **about 9:30 p.m.**, we heard the band from the pub next door come back from a break, waking us up. We talked and laughed about the music. Dale even asked if I knew the artist when they played "Spirit in the Sky" (Norman Greenbaum). Then he took another 800 mg Ibuprofen™ as the headache was better but not gone, and got up to use the bathroom. That was normal. He even asked to leave the light on in the bathroom as a nightlight, walked to bed, and must have *fallen* into it because he knocked into me hard, and it was a king bed. I teased him to stay on his own side but got no reply. **He was gone**—*vacant eyes, jerky movements, no speech, putting his mouthpiece in askew.* I turned on the light. He didn't answer to know his name or mine, couldn't put his hands up in the air when I asked, and when I said, "let's lie down," he sat straight up and touched his toes. ***Scary...***

> *I'm recognizing more and yielding to patience and listening to precious Holy Spirit; His timing, not mine. God knows exactly where we are with all this, and He is faithful to lead.*

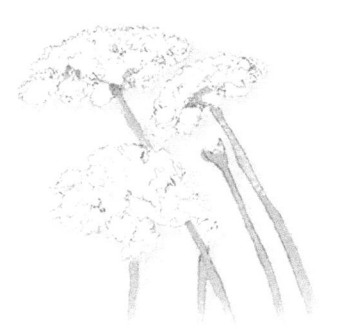

I called 911 but had no cell service on the island, so went to the porch and saw the employee who checked us in, told him to "call 911, that my call didn't go through, and my husband was having a stroke." The owners came to stay with me until the ambulance arrived. EMT said I could ride up front, so I called my kids until the EMT came back and said they were going to airflight Dale to UF Health in Jacksonville. I packed our bag, got my GPS ready, and headed out alone for the hour drive to the hospital, talking to my kids on the way there, knowing Nancy and Ken were already on the road from North Carolina to be with me.

Chapter Two

THE FIRST MONTH

10/4/14 – In the Wee Hours of the Morning – First Caring Bridge Entry

Dear friends,
There's no easy way to tell you that at **10:00 p.m. Oct. 3rd (last night)** Dale had a stroke. We were at Amelia Island (on our way to Hilton Head for a vacation to be followed by Dale's forty-five-year Gator football team reunion) and we were awake in bed listening to a neighboring pub band playing oldies. During a break in the music, Dale went into the bathroom before we went to sleep and when he returned, he actually <u>fell</u> onto the bed, no longer functioning normally. Fortunately, I was awake and immediately noticed the symptoms so was able to call 911 within two minutes. Paramedics confirmed the likelihood of a stroke and flew him to UF Health Jacksonville while I followed, guided by GPS, and arrived just as the ER doctor was calling me. On her expert and personal advice, they administered tPA (tissue Plasminogen Activator) for acute ischemic stroke just at two hours from onset and Dale was moved to SICU about 4:30 a.m.

The medical staff has been wonderful; Dale's confusion and frustration is great, but he did improve after the tPA and, after MUCH agitation, slept most of this morning. As of last report at 4:30 a.m., he is neither communicating nor understanding commands; his right side is gravely affected/paralyzed but movement has continued to return to his right arm and leg.

My sister Nancy and brother-in-law Ken were with me by 3:00 a.m. and Christy, David, and Stephanie are on their way now. I will have family with me during our stay in Jacksonville and hope to move Dale closer to home very soon. Can't yet think much farther ahead.

Only God knows the outcome and His Presence, leading, and wisdom have been evident to me. I am blessed that when Dale was stricken, he wasn't driving, wasn't alone, that our new insurance was in place, and that his complete medical history had been updated that morning as a travel prep and we had it with us. I trust God to lead my steps and will follow one step at a time. (This afternoon my first step was to get some sleep.)

"For I know the plans I have for you," declares the LORD, "plans to prosper you and not to harm you, plans to give you hope and a future."   *Jeremiah 29:11 (NIV)*

"I know not what the future holds, but I know Who holds the future..."

9:00 A.M.

Upon waking, I spoke with today's nurse. Dale was fully conscious this morning, not on any meds and no restraints. He is doing well with understanding but struggling to say something to her. She tried all the obvious—bathroom, pain, hot/cold...no success. He has his glasses on and I told her to put ESPN™ on the TV as it's his high interest, and to tell him that his wife and kids will be there soon. They brushed his teeth; he has a slight droop on the left side so can't hold water in his mouth or gargle. He's resting well—**all good news.** We're on our way over now after a good night's sleep.

> **NOTE: In meeting with the doctor that first morning, the MRI showed 3 strokes - 2 new ones and 1 old one. I told him there was "no old stroke" and gave him the brain**

MRI from 2013 (which showed NO stroke). I then realized that the changes we noted in September must have come from a lesser stroke, we just weren't aware of the stroke event happening. (See 10/3/14 entry, 8:00 p.m. Amelia Island)

> *"I know not what the future holds, but I know Who holds the future..."*

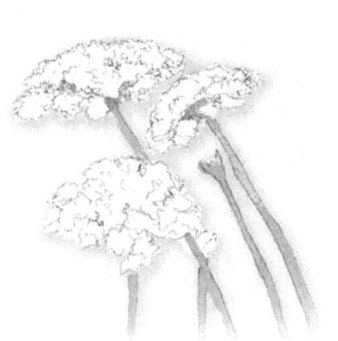

10/5/14 - ICU

All good news today. Dale sat in a chair most of the day; his understanding is good, and sense of humor is back. It's now a guessing game for communication, although he is making sounds and few words—I, who—and many gestures, motions. It is frustrating for us all, but he's determined to make it work and has a great attitude for which we are thankful. He is trying many ways to write and point things out. His sight is still impaired, but his right hand is strong and active, and his dexterity improved during the day. He will be moved out of ICU tonight and therapies start tomorrow. I will meet with the case manager tomorrow to find a rehab facility close to home. Please pray for guidance with that and an available room.

The weather was beautiful today and we got to enjoy the outdoors some since only two of us could be with him at a time in ICU. David and Christy watched football with him while Steph and I were able to enjoy some time outside at the Jacksonville riverfront. I am so thankful for fresh air and beauty. We are blessed!

10/6/14 – Up and Down Day

Very hard night for Dale. Didn't sleep much at all after he was awakened for vitals check. (Consequently, his roommate hardly got any sleep either.)

Was **very** disoriented and scared and, since he still has great strength with poor vision and little understanding, they had to use restraints on him for his safety. ***VERY hard.*** Dale is still unable to communicate, and extremely agitated by that as you can imagine. I got here at 7:00 a.m. and he's resting now, thankfully. I am waiting for the doctors and case manager. Prayers are greatly appreciated; your encouraging words bring refreshing.

Evening Update

It's been an up and down day. Dale is exhibiting great frustration with trying to communicate interspersed with a sweet, short visit from a dear friend who lives locally—prayer and *latte*—and a surprise visit from Dale's cousin Keith who drove up from Orlando. Keith came at a difficult time and got a reality check of the trauma we face. My sister Carol arrived to stay over with me; her patience, experience, and prayer are a treasure. Dale was standing up when she arrived, so she got a real hug!

Other than the huge communication issues, his physical improvements are outstanding! He walked all around the neuro floor with just someone near him and followed commands well, went to the bathroom himself, and washed/dried hands at the sink. We met with physical, occupational, and speech therapists for evaluation. Dale needs work on manual dexterity and wants to write, but it's not happening yet with his right hand. He had his first soft food meal and tries to eat by himself, but that needs to improve; he did drink alone from a glass. There will be lots of speech therapy needed as the stroke was dead center in the Broca's area, the language center.

The attending doctor said he can be released to a rehab facility as early as tomorrow, so we are looking close to home; all suggestions are appreciated. Please pray that he has a good night's sleep, peace and patience, and continued restoration.

NOTE: There is SO much I wish I knew then. So I share a few practical helps now from what I've learned since, in no particular order, simply for you to consider as soon as possible. This is in no way medical advice, simply lessons learned from a caregiving life. And, of course, every situation and person is unique so you must consider what could work in your caregiving:

-A traumatic brain injury, including stroke or concussion causes the brain to swell so any part that is affected by the event can provoke behavior, thinking and speech that is highly abnormal for that individual, but they personally are not likely to realize it at first.

-Brain energy is quickly depleted due to much energy being used for the healing process.

-Any type of stimulation can quickly become overwhelming, especially sight and light. We later learned from a vision therapist that 70% of brain energy is directed to sight and light…through the eyes. Therefore, a "brain break" with a blackout eye mask for 20 minutes or so gives the brain the best rest – no sight or light; quiet helps as well. Look for signs of anxiety or tiredness and take a brain break immediately. This can be done on a regular basis almost anytime in the

hospital...and later in the car or at home. Keep a good eye mask with you everywhere and keep a watchful eye out for when a brain break is needed.

-Consider how you would like to be treated if in this traumatic situation yourself. The reality can sometimes be that you would want those helping you to make the best possible decision when you are not able to, hard though that may be for you as a caregiver.

-Kindness and consideration are always helpful.

-Simplify decisions. Give choices of either/or, applesauce or yogurt, eggs or oatmeal, red or yellow; not "what do you want to eat?"

-Take things slowly; pause when needed; take deep breaths and encourage them to as well.

-PRESENCE is IMPORTANT, peaceful presence. Just being there, knowing someone cares and they are not alone is very calming and promotes healing. Anything anxiety-producing causes energy to be spent on the anxiety instead of on healing.

-If touch is not painful or anxiety-producing, skin to skin contact can be a comfort: holding hands, touching the arm or leg, hand on the brow. Also consider a cool or warm cloth on the forehead or eyes, brushing hair, lightly massaging hands, arms, legs, or feet.

-Play familiar or calming music, music they like, and encourage singing or humming. Even humming stimulates the vagus nerve that works directly with the vital organs. Individuals can often hum or sing to some degree even if they can't speak.

-Consider beauty and order and how it can help with visual calming, especially in an unfamiliar place.

-Bring printed copies or large pictures of individual family members, favorite people and pets to display on a wall that they can see from their bed. If speech is impaired, put an identifying and/or relationship name under each photo so others in the room can converse about the pictures and relationships.

-Speak life, truth, and hope aloud. Positive statements or happenings. Laugh! Collect jokes and read them aloud. Watch funny videos or comedy routines, old or new.

-Verbalize things you are thankful for and encourage everyone to do so. Every day. Consider keeping a thankfulness/gratitude journal – daily list just 3 things for which you can be thankful; that way you can revisit the positive and count your blessings.

-Give the gift of anticipation, something to look forward to: food from outside the hospital, phone call or FaceTime with a friend, going outside on a sunny day, new pictures.

-Prepare for rehab and restoration to be a marathon, not a 5K, as it takes time for the brain swelling to subside, for connections to be restored, and/or new neural pathways to form. But the brain is always changing…which always brings hope.

10/7/14 – From David

"Quick update on my Dad. His recovery is going well, and he is showing great improvement in his physical movement. He is able to get up and walk on his own as well as drink on his own. Food is still a challenge by himself, but swallowing is no problem. Communication is still the number one obstacle as he still can't speak or write. He has started to form some words, but it is very frustrating for all. We are working with the case manager to move him to an acute rehab facility in the next forty-eight hours closer to home. He will be there until communication and function allow him to be home. We look forward to that day and appreciate the prayers! Mom is dealing well, but it has been very hard because of the lack of communication. Thank you all for the kind words and advice!"

10/8/14 – Moving to Rehab in Sarasota

We made it through the night without incident, thankfully, although restless. Spent most of the day waiting for paperwork to be done for discharge. Dale walked a lot, was awake most of the day, ate very well, drank from a cup with his right/weak hand, and was very happy for Christy's volleyball team's victory over Charlotte High School!

We are leaving now for the rehab facility in Sarasota where he will be for at least a week, with further evaluation at that point. I will make trips home and be staying with my sister Patti and her husband Bill in Sarasota. My brother Rick and sister-in-law Melodie also live there and we'll only be forty-five minutes from home and David, Stephanie, and the boys. Dale's sister Kim and her husband Kevin plan to come down first thing tomorrow and Nancy and Ken will visit again before heading north. Dale was VERY excited to be moving on to rehab! The anticipation could be felt by everyone.

We are so grateful for all of those who helped us at UF Health Jacksonville, for all of your prayers and encouragement, and the advice of those who have been through this experience. We know there's a long road ahead of us and are grateful for this next step.

To God be the glory!

IMPORTANT NOTE REGARDING TRANSPORT: At this point, I knew NOTHING about medical practices and Dale experienced great trauma on the trip and reception at the new rehab, much of which could have been avoided if I had known how to prepare, what to ask, and TO ASSUME NOTHING. In my ignorance, I <u>expected</u> the attendants would be told what his needs were and what to do for him; I <u>assumed</u> those on the receiving end would also have been told what his needs were and what to do for him. THEY DID NOT! THEY DID NOT!!! The medical charts/info may have given the basic info, but <u>you can NEVER assume</u> that medical personnel of any caliber have the time to read carefully, or understand the depth of the devastation, especially in "fresh" trauma.

Dale was not fed or toileted during the entire four-hour trip. He couldn't speak or assess his needs, although he was totally conscious the whole time. I was following the transport but lost actual sight of them when I stopped to get gas and was not there to meet Dale when he arrived at the new rehab facility. The timing was <u>awful</u>. It was during a shift change, and Dale was left sitting in front of the nurse's station strapped into a wheelchair with no one he knew, unable to communicate, not having been fed or toileted. The admitting staff was not readily available due to the shift change and when I arrived; he was in full view of them but with nothing having been done. I was shocked and furious... but had to tend to that later.

Immediately I was at his side comforting him, vocalizing his needs loudly, and giving him something to eat and drink. The staff did help me then and I called both David and my brother who lived nearby who came immediately for encouragement and support for us both while we got him settled in his room. It took several hours for Dale to even relax. Plus, unbeknownst to us, his own expectations had not been totally realistic; he knew he was leaving the hospital, but this new place looked and sounded like a hospital and he thought we had lied to him. He really only relaxed and slept when I climbed onto his bed with him and slept next to him that night, all night.

I would NEVER again allow that situation to arise for a patient who isn't able to communicate for himself or on medication that impaired his understanding. That is my sole reason for sharing this scenario here, for the reader's readiness. I was still traumatized myself, tired and totally ignorant of how to prepare for this. You are now informed. God be with you.

Any future transports were handled with the following:
　-A close family member was on hand to meet the transport in case something happened to me en route.
　-I understood/confirmed all meds, meals and toilet needs with transport staff, gave them my name/phone number and that of the other family member.
　-I briefed them on his communication issues and how to best communicate with him.
　-Dale's name and my name and phone number were on a lanyard around his neck.
　-I gave them a personal info sheet written out that told them personal info about Dale including his full name, age, where he lives and grew up, career and interests,

wife's name, kids and grandkids' names/ages, goals to recovery... anything that could be a touch point for conversation during transport.

10/9/14 – Dale's 64th Birthday

This sure has turned our world upside down. After a long ride and rough transition upon arrival at Sarasota facility, I stayed over with Dale as he settled in. Well, we never expected his 64th birthday would be his first full day at the rehab center. The staff here had "Happy Birthday Dale" signs up and gave him orange and blue balloons, fully recognizing his UF Gator connection! He had visits from David, Nancy and Ken, Kim and Kevin, and Patti. He had a great day at therapy throughout the day and night, and I actually got to meet all of the key people that will be working with him, a great success. Communication is the primary focus here; physically Dale has his strength back and walks extremely well. They are working to improve overall coordination. Evaluations took place in physical therapy, occupational therapy, and speech therapy today. Night was hard once again and he began to respond better to the staff here than he would for me, so I left to spend the night with Patti and Bill, who thankfully live close by.

10/10/14 – Learning More – Homonymous Hemianopsia

Well, adjusting is very hard for Dale and communication is still SO slow, to the point that at times we have to give it up for the moment, revisiting it later as needed. A former student wrote to tell us of her stroke insights from when she stroked *during high school:* she first thought her speech was just fine and *everyone else was just not getting it*! After a while she realized **her** speech was what had changed. Dale recently came to that realization, which has led to much less striving, waiting until he's calm and relaxed. We are learning things we wish we'd known; for example, "sundowners" is new info for me, yet it appears that is happening as Dale's evenings have been more confused and agitated.

Let me say very candidly that this is all extremely hard for Dale and for all of us in the family.

Dale's eyesight is highly abnormal—homonymous hemianopsia (HH)—loss of half the visual field of view in the same side of both eyes. In his case, the right side. He is very physically strong, but eyesight affects coordination; actually, *it affects everything*. He can't see the TV or read; his depth perception is terrible as he goes to eat or walk or move, and he grabs at shadows on the floor. My #1 prayer is for improvement in that area.

From the Eyes of the Beholder
HOW VISUAL FIELD CUTS MAY APPEAR TO STROKE SURVIVORS

Communication is basically based on how we can work through the struggle together. If he's calm, he hears well and has good comprehension... unless he has to think through multiple steps. Asking questions with Yes/No answers is best for now and Dale uses gestures as he can; however, the speech therapists (SLPs) want him to try to speak the words as well as use gestures. We are playing music in his room nearly all the time for enjoyment and **brain engagement**. Dale's response is notable—singing as he can, rhythm, humming, air guitar...or peacefulness when listening to quiet music.

I will not be staying overnight any more now that he is responding to the staff, and I have met everyone involved. *I was becoming overwhelmed and am conscious of the need for me to stay rested and healthy.* I have confidence that this staff is knowledgeable and doing everything in Dale's best interests... even if it's hard.

I had an informative meeting with his doctor this morning, very experienced. He believes this facility is the best in the state for Dale. The staff will walk him when restless, but they will not restrain him, and for that we are grateful. The main goal is to keep Dale safe, so he has a wander guard on his leg, basically confining him to this floor; an alarm would go off if he were to open a door or the elevator.

I had to feed him more today than yesterday, his left eye is somewhat sore, and both eyes were red. Don't know if that's from lack of sleep or not but they are going to look at his left eye tonight and treat it as needed. Focus is on getting his days/nights straightened out and changing medication accordingly. Seems like his therapies went fine but he didn't have much response when I asked him.

He was very excited to be able to go outside tonight and spent a lot of time looking out the window before David arrived with his whole family. We went downstairs to a Classic Car Show held right at the facility's parking lot. After walking the entire car show, Dale was very tired from all the various stimuli and asked for the wheelchair, so we all went into the day room and the kids played the piano for us. Patti and Bill came for a visit as well.

I went home to my own house, spent time talking with our grandsons about Papa and answering their questions after they had seen him. I have to say that David's explanation of brain injury was *inspired* and good for the boys. Joshua spent the night with me to help unload my car and get our "vacation" things out of it. I got somewhat settled and will pack a bag to stay the weekend, sleeping at Patti's and going to my house occasionally. It's been very different for me to eat meals out regularly, but it sure has been a blessing when family/visitors bring me healthy, easy food. Lots of changes...

Let me end by saying how much your love and words are helpful to us all, including Dale. The other night as I read them he was totally engaged, interacting with me about many people and incidents. It was precious. You are greatly loved by us, and I thank you from the bottom of my heart for keeping up with us and for praying.

10/11/14 – Saturday...

On Saturday, the therapies are not routine, but Dale had been scheduled for several in the morning. I had been at home and gathered more appropriate clothes for Dale, a few days' worth for me, and paid some bills. I arrived after his sessions and he was napping, then helped him with lunch. With no scheduled events for the rest of the day, we "watched" the Texas/Oklahoma game, being big fans of both coaches Bob Stoops and Charlie Strong. We had a nice visit with a longtime friend and then made some new friends in the day room here. Later, we read some notes from all our wonderful friends and supporters. They are much appreciated, especially today since Dale was greatly saddened to miss his 45th Gator football team reunion this weekend... but was proudly wearing all his Gator gear!

10/12/14 – Christy Visit and Art

Dale had a bad night and it started just before I left around 7:30 p.m. He didn't sleep well, so this morning he was sleeping for several hours after a couple of therapies. Christy and a dear friend visited on their way back from Gainesville with lots of news about Gators and volleyball. That was SO good for Dale! Christy's team got #1 seed for districts and get to play on home court! Mid-afternoon, the art therapist came into the day room to find Dale and he focused on art for over an hour! I never would have expected him to engage in that, but he's been trying to write and communicate through drawing.

I'm learning lots from a book recommended by my sister's friend, *A Stroke Of Insight* by Jill Bolte Taylor, a neuroscientist who had a stroke at age thirty-four. I am so thankful for technology that I can text and gather information and communicate with others without disturbing Dale's rest or raising questions. God is good...

10/13/14 – My Job as Dale's Advocate

Got behind with entries... much to do. We think Dale's night meds have had a paradoxical effect, producing a result the opposite of what was intended, so he really needs rest—to heal, to do therapy well, and to stay clearheaded. My day was filled with meetings—day nurse, case manager, day supervisor—and making lists for tomorrow's meetings. Kim and her daughter Kate arrived before me at the end of Dale's therapies (which went well) and he actually played ball with them at PT. Kim said he ate well by himself, but didn't eat much. He never did settle down this afternoon, but was overstimulated, likely because of lack of sleep. Afternoon therapies went very well also, and Kim and Kate were there to attend meetings with me. It was eye-opening to say the least; we asked many questions and also learned much. The meetings were very productive, and changes were initiated; they changed some procedures, made everyone aware of HH eye issue and Dale's <u>need</u> for his glasses, and his doctor ordered a different, stronger sedative.

I cannot stress enough how I believe every patient whose thinking is impaired by trauma, illness, or medication needs an advocate. Having been with each of my parents as they were hospitalized and with Dale through surgeries, I find both patient and staff benefit from having someone with the patient regularly; it helps to keep things running smoothly. That's my free advice! You're all giving so much to us; we'll give back what we can.

Progress:
- basically eating alone with spoon in right hand
- washes face and hands and brushes teeth alone
- watched SportCenter™ and really engaged with it once he sat in the day room across the room from a larger TV.

10/14/14 - Much Work to Do

Good news! Dale slept through the entire night! He was peaceful this morning waiting to go to therapy. He also ate breakfast and lunch himself; I just need to stay out of the way (I'm learning). He rested after lunch with his eyes closed. I met with neurologist, psychologist, PT, OT, and SLP. Basically, although restoration can continue for years, the majority of motor recovery is within three months, speech improves slowly and longer mainly over six to nine months, and sight with Homonymous Hemianopsia (HH), if it's going to improve, within a month or two. Neurologist said personally he has only seen one patient recover from HH. I am pursuing light therapy and info on prism glasses. Therapists all say he works very hard. PT practices stairs with him since at our home we have four steps just eight feet outside our front door and Dale needs more confidence going down; OT working on recovering dexterity in his right hand (Dale is right-handed), and the SLP has the most work to do with communication, eating, and cognition. All have to teach him how to compensate for HH issues.

Progress:
- night meds are helping Dale get the rest he needs
- handles his personal hygiene when cued and with minimal assistance (struggles to locate toothbrush, faucets, soap)
- identified simple pictures correctly when given two choices
- makes the *M* sound
- located an orange spoon more easily when eating than standard silverware but we're still not sure how he is processing colors.

I read more of your personal notes to him; please keep them coming and *address them specifically to him.* He is listening attentively and it's a great exercise in remembering people and events as well as receiving love and positive encouragement. Any cards received are posted on the wall and he *loves* pointing them out to everyone.

10/15/14 – Baby Steps

Had a good night but was awake till nearly midnight so doctor ordered ALL meds and vitals to be completed by 6:30 p.m. so when Dale winds down, there's no further disturbance. Dale had a great therapy day, but he was tired by lunch and sleepy for afternoon therapy. I scheduled an appointment with neuro ophthalmologist for next Tuesday to determine the extent of his visual field cuts and identify the location. It appears that he sees in the upper right quadrant of both eyes so they're working to have him scan to the right and lower his chin to see more. I got a team report from the case manager, and it was good; I then met with SLP, PT and doctor.

Dale is visibly moved by reading your personal notes and we often add memories of our own. Please pray regarding next steps; he is only approved here for ten days and insurance approves what happens next based on progress reports.

Progress:
- needs only stand-by assistance (SBA) for showering, brushing teeth, getting dressed
- got elastic shoelaces
- psychologist encouraged him and also determined he can ID colors correctly
- initiated singing a song when he heard it - carries a tune well (glad that's still normal as music is so important to him)
- *doctor released him to go outside with family - yay!*

My sister Carol arrived for a few days, and we plan to take him outside in the morning.

10/16/14 - A Day Off for Me

Today was an interesting day. Dale slept through the night and had a therapy session at 8:30 a.m. Carol and I took him outside for about twenty minutes for the very first time, then more therapies throughout the day. She is so wonderful with Dale, having been through surgery/brain injury with her husband Steve and through extensive hand and wrist rehab herself. So, I had a day off and Carol went to therapies with him, had lunch, worked on hand exercises, and did art together. They drew the pond we saw in the morning; he recognized her gator and added "blue sky" to her drawing. It was a very good day yet exhausting.

I caught up on phone calls, took a nap, had a great visit with family friends and their kids at the park for about forty-five minutes this afternoon. It was great therapy for me—fresh air, sunshine, sweet conversation, smiling faces, children playing with their dad on the playground, and even a three-month-old smiling baby in my lap for the entire visit! Loved it and them. Then a massage from my sister-in-law, Melodie. Wonderful day for me as well.

Progress:
- counting aloud in PT
- socializing purposefully
- very gently played ball with frail older woman in wheelchair
- working hard in speech - repeating sounds/words much more clearly
- eating more
- singing along with songs
- clapping for himself and others for PT successes
- since Dale recognizes color, I've applied bright orange duct tape to the right side of his meal tray, faucets and other items. Immediately effective to assist in scanning to the right.

10/17/14 - Neuro Ophthalmologist Appointment

Great news! God blessed us with the perfect answer for getting Dale to the eye doctor's this morning. Last night, Carol and I were discussing how Dale would respond to going off campus and then having to return. I decided to ask for someone "official" to bring him to the car and meet us when we returned. Just before bedtime, I was reminded to call Dale's new friend on staff here at the rehab so when I reached him this morning to ask for help to get Dale into the car to go to the doctor's appointment, he asked why the facility wasn't transporting him. Well, the truth is I didn't know they could or would, and his doctor had said we could take him ourselves. So, this wonderful man made the decision that the rehab would transport Dale and that Carol and I could ride along as well. We are thrilled with this because we did have questions about how Dale would feel about coming back to the rehab after having some freedom. This way he'll be with "official" personnel and we're not in charge. All glory to God Who is watching over us, leading us step-by-step and giving us favor with others.

As it turned out, at the appointment Dale was not able to follow the more complex directions for taking field of vision test so ophthalmologist can't tell vision details yet. The good news is that his eyes have full mobility, are symmetrical and healthy, physiologically not affected by the stroke. We have another appointment in two weeks to try again.

I had meetings most of the rest of the day and worked on phone calls for next step of therapy so here's Carol's report on therapy:
    -pretended to use a steering wheel to drive his wheelchair down the hall - just for fun
    -throwing a ball back and forth to me while balancing on a balance board - very impressive
    -recognized shapes

- picked out his name when given a choice of printed names in large letters - DALE or BOB
- associated orange color card with me by pointing to my shirt
- followed sequential commands correctly and quickly - touch shoulder, nose, foot, etc.
- followed therapist over set of orange and yellow rings spaced on floor, stepping over and balancing on one foot - only difficulty was with rings outside of his field of vision.

Got word that insurance extended Dale's stay until Thursday, October 23rd. I will appeal for further extension on Monday as his doctor would like him to stay as inpatient to continue aggressive therapy in cognitive, speech, and dexterity since those areas are so greatly affected by the visual impairment.

10/18/14 - Thriving After Rest

It is amazing what rest can do! Four solid nights' sleep this week and Dale's thriving. No therapies scheduled for today so when Carol and I arrived today, he'd been bored and was in the day room studying large dominoes and jigsaw puzzles. He matched a few dominoes, then after Carol left, he had lunch and I noticed much-improved right-side function, now after two weeks, and he doesn't want help. He's off Risperdal as of last night and is much more cognitive today, scanning better to right side, too. I will be interested to see the therapists' evaluations on Monday.

Family friends came by today for a visit; they were my parents' best friends. They played tic-tac-toe with Dale, shared encouragement, and prayed with us. Another friend brought me lunch and, after Dale woke up from a nap, the three of us went outside on this beautiful day to sit across from the lake for about an hour, socializing with everyone who came out there. Dale went with our friend to help a guy in a wheelchair up the incline sidewalk, very sweet. We came in to actually watch some football on TV; his vision seems much improved today or at least he's finding things on the right side more easily. That is very encouraging. After dinner, we worked with the dominoes again and helped turn over jigsaw pieces for another patient. Dale really wanted to watch the Gator game, but it wasn't on the rehab TV and he didn't just want to listen to audio - *sad*.

I pray that with the change in meds and no Risperdal in his system that he will still sleep well.

Progress:
- alert, engaged
- sought out things to do on his own
- looked through magazine without frustration
- used children's book to ID numbers and read some words
- hugged spontaneously
- very appreciative

Book: My Stroke of Insight

I recently sent my family a copy of a book that was suggested to us after Dale's stroke, very helpful to me in understanding stroke and brain injury and recovery.

"My Stroke of Insight" by Jill Bolte Taylor, is the story of a brain scientist who had and recovered from a stroke, relating how she felt and what helped her while recovering. *"I wanted to communicate: 'Yelling louder does not help me understand you any better! Don't be afraid of me. Come closer to me. Bring me your gentle spirit. Speak more slowly. Enunciate more clearly. Again! Please, try again! S-l-o-w down. Be kind to me. Be a safe place for me. See that I am a wounded animal, not a stupid animal. I am vulnerable and* *confused. Whatever my age, whatever my credentials, reach for me. Respect me. I am in here. Come find me.'"*[1]

Many of us have never been up *close and personal* with someone who has suffered a stroke. I'm learning so much and will guard Dale's energy and time so he can heal and have energy for his new job: recovering. *As much as we need and appreciate visits, I and my children would ask that you read several sections that are particularly enlightening before you visit,* especially the list included below (it's an Appendix from the book), available on Amazon or at your library. *Please read Chapter Nine "Day Two: The Morning After."* Chapters two and three are also very informational and helpful in understanding brain function and what happens during and after a brain trauma.

Forty Things I Need the Most: (from "My Stroke of Insight" by Jill Bolte Taylor)

1. I am not stupid, I am wounded. Please respect me.
2. Come close, speak slowly, and enunciate clearly.
3. Repeat yourself - assume I know nothing and start from the beginning, over and over.
4. Be as patient with me the 20th time you teach me something, as you were the first.
5. Approach me with an open heart and slow your energy down. Take your time.
6. Be aware of what your body language and facial expressions are communicating to me.
7. Make eye contact with me. I am in here – come find me. Encourage me.
8. Please don't raise your voice – I'm not deaf, I'm wounded.
9. Touch me appropriately and connect with me.

---

[1] (Taylor, My Stroke of Insight 2006)

10. Honor the healing power of sleep.
11. Protect my energy. No talk radio, TV, or nervous visitors! Keep visitation brief (five minutes).
12. Stimulate my brain when I have any energy to learn something new, but know that a small amount may wear me out quickly.
13. Use age-appropriate (toddler) educational toys and books to teach me.
14. Introduce me to the world kinesthetically. Let me feel everything. (I am an infant again.)
15. Teach me with monkey-see, monkey-do behavior.
16. Trust that I am trying – just not with your skill level or on your schedule.
17. Ask me multiple-choice questions. Avoid Yes/No questions.
18. Ask me questions with specific answers. Allow me time to hunt for an answer.
19. Do not assess my cognitive ability by how fast I can think.
20. Handle me gently, as you would handle a newborn.
21. Speak to me directly, not about me to others.
22. Cheer me on. Expect me to recover completely, even if it takes twenty years!
23. Trust that my brain can always continue to learn.
24. Break all actions down into smaller steps of action.
25. Look for what obstacles prevent me from succeeding on a task.
26. Clarify for me what the next level or step is so I know what I am working toward.
27. Remember that I have to be proficient at one level of function before I can move on to the next level.
28. Celebrate all of my little successes. They inspire me.
29. Please don't finish my sentences for me or fill in words I can't find. I need to work my brain.
30. If I can't find an old file, make it a point to create a new one.
31. I may want you to think I understand more than I really do.

32. Focus on what I can do rather than bemoan what I cannot do.
33. Introduce me to my old life. Don't assume that because I cannot play like I used to play that I won't continue to enjoy music or an instrument, etc.
34. Remember that in the absence of some functions, I have gained other abilities.
35. Keep me familiar with my family, friends, and loving support. Build a collage wall of cards and photos that I can see. Label them so I can review them.
36. Call in the troops! Create a healing team for me. Send word out to everyone so they can send me love. Keep them abreast of my condition and ask them to do specific things to support me – like visualize me being able to swallow with ease or rocking my body up into a sitting position.
37. Love me for who I am today. Don't hold me to being the person I was before. I have a different brain now.
38. Be protective of me but do not stand in the way of my progress.
39. Show me old video footage of me doing things to remind me about how I spoke, walked, and gestured.
40. Remember that my medications probably make me feel tired, as well as mask my ability to know what it feels like to be me.

10/19/14 - Up & Down Day

An up and down day. Dale didn't rest as well after his first day off Risperdal. Went to sleep last night about 8:30 p.m. (when he'd been asleep by 7:00 p.m. for five nights); then he was restless around 3:30 a.m. and up for good at 4:30 a.m. (when he had been waking at 6:30 a.m.) That seemed to affect his clarity all day and he had several hours of weepiness. Although I understand that ups and downs are part of the recovery process, I was not prepared for the big change from yesterday, so I was emotionally affected myself.

We had a sweet and timely visit from Christy and her best friend who is like another daughter to us. Dale got caught up with Christy's Gulf Coast volleyball team, Gator football, and GCHS golf team. Both the girls set up new playlists on Spotify according to Dale's likes, and we sang several songs together. He played a lot of air guitar but has yet to pick up the guitar I brought from home a few days ago. We walked a good distance outside, too. After lunch, David visited with two of his boys. We all played catch in the dayroom and could see the familiar "Papa" as he threw the ball. Then went to the PT room and David went through many of the therapy exercises with him so he could personally gauge Dale's physicality, so Dale got in an extra PT session! Papa then read out loud along with the boys from Dr. Seuss; he used very good expression and vocalizing but it saddened him after a while. Together, we put up a family picture wall from pics Stephanie had printed out. Art therapy was mid-afternoon; the teacher brought Motown music, so they drew to that. She is wonderful and upbeat and very caring; came to the room to share personal stories and inspiration.

Dale was exhausted by 5:00 p.m. and fell asleep in the chair. He had night meds at 6:00 p.m. and they settled him in for the night. I moved in for a stay with my friend in Sarasota this evening; we are all so grateful for the love and care we are receiving.

Progress:
- coordinated movement in throwing/catching ball
- moves head to scan to right more naturally
- drinking lots of water
- vocalization is more pronounced
- positive reactions to music; great recall of artists he likes.

October 3, 2014 was a milestone, an altar, a turning point, an end, a beginning, yet a next simple step in hearing from the One Who leads and guides our path. For decades I've trusted Him, God, my Daddy, Jesus, my Lord and Savior, my Comforter and Teacher, Holy Spirit.

I've sung and ministered Twila Paris's song "Do I Trust You?" with integrity of heart and standing on the Rock, yet here it comes to me again tonight playing in my mind as I begin to journal. Do I trust Him? My answer - an unequivocal YES.

10/20-21/14 - Crisis... and Resolution

Were in crisis yesterday, the 20th. Dale got very little sleep, and consequently, little clarity or understanding during the day. His therapy sessions were futile. He had acupuncture and rested a short time, more peaceable for a while but overtired and overwhelmed. Dale retired at 6:30 p.m. although the doctor wanted him awake until meds at 9:00 p.m. I went home and was called after Dale woke up around 10:00 p.m. and he became agitated, confused, and a definite danger to himself and others because of his fear, strength, and lack of understanding. He was taken to Sarasota Memorial (SMH) under the Baker Act. I did not go back up to Sarasota as David was there with Dale. He and my sister Patti spent the night with him peacefully, first in the ER, then in his room after he was admitted to SMH for testing.

I came up early and spent today with him, meeting new doctors and going through evaluations. The staff was impressed with the records from UF Health in Jacksonville; we learned that his echocardiogram was clean, but also of a **Prothrombin 20210 gene mutation in his blood, an inherited condition that increases one's predisposition to develop abnormal blood clots.** They did another CT scan ruling out a bleed and an MRI to compare with one dated October 4th. Tomorrow, he'll have a transesophageal echocardiogram (TEE) hoping to find a source of the clots. (both MRIs - October 4th and today showed two new strokes and one 'old' one since approximately October 2013).

I am very impressed with all the staff at SMH and quality of care and response. Although this is such a hard time as Dale has still had little sleep for three nights now, we know he's in good hands and expect that rest and medical plans will assist in his restoration.

Bright spots in these two days:
- visits from our pastors
- brother-in-law Bill's research
- our son David, a godly man and honorable son
- police officer's compassionate care of Dale and our family
- Patti's availability and, of course, love and good food
- visit from friends and offers of help when we return home
- today's technology keeping family and info at our fingertips
- those who've walked this walk sharing insight, hope and their stories
- smiling, caring, knowledgeable medical staff
- my dear friend having laundered Dale's clothes
- Christy's GCHS Sharks' volleyball team winning first round of districts.

10/22/14 – New Storm, Same Rock

Well, the day started peaceably although Dale slept a total of 6 ½ hours. He was comfortable in his surroundings and took direction well. Nothing by mouth since midnight (NPO, I've learned) so I just rested on the bed with him until OT came in for evaluation. Then he left for the TEE, and I met with doctors and discussed med changes and their long-range plan for him. Afterwards Dale had a late lunch, we rested awhile and shared about visitors, volleyball, and the TEE results which were clear; his heart is healthy inside and out. Not really surprising, but definitely good news.

By 2:30 p.m., however, we were in trauma; Dale was restless, overstimulated, then **extremely** agitated and confused. I stepped out of the room to let the professionals minister to him and it took several strong and experienced individuals to attend to him. Although this situation was *VERY* difficult to for me to observe and for the staff to employ, they utilized every means available to them...*with my permission*...including a Posey bed.

Dale was exhausted—physically, mentally, and emotionally depleted, continually distraught, and really never settled or rested before I left at 7:30 p.m., even with medication. I had been in and out of his room as he had periods of responding to me and times he was more responsive to those in uniform. This staff on the neuro floor is WONDERFUL and Dale is right where he should be, *with people who understand his needs as a brain-injured patient.* (This was fittingly compared to those who work with ESE students—*least restrictive environment with safety for both him and those around him.*) Doctor's orders include having someone in the room with him at all times, plus they wisely located his room directly next the nursing station. I left for the night after meeting the night staff and telling Dale about my plans to get some sleep and see him in the morning and my trust in this hospital staff. ***Might be the hardest day I've ever had, certainly the most emotional.***

We are not having visitors right now while they work to find the best means to help Dale stabilize. We've never been at a place like this before—me, Dale, or our kids. This is a new storm but the same Rock we've stood on for most of our lives.

"The rain came down the streams rose, and the winds blew and beat against that house; yet it did not fall, because it had its foundation on the rock"
Matthew 7:24-27

"The Lord is my rock, my fortress and my deliverer...in whom I take refuge"
Psalm 18:2

"For who is God besides the LORD? and who is the Rock besides our God?"   Psalm 18:31

Today's blessings:
- quiet morning talk with Dale just lying on his bed
- good and positive test results as medical staff search for source of the strokes
- doctors who hug, smile and give thorough explanations
- Melodie's gift of lunch and a visit
- kind, tenderhearted, wise hospital staff and their care for us.
- a visit from our rabbi friend and his wife whom we've known since our daughters were seated next to each other in middle school, then became best friends and college roomies. More later on their words of wisdom.
- texting - what a blessed way of communicating in the quiet
- Patti's delicious dinner and conversation about her trip (not hospital talk)
- nurses and staff that bless us and pray for us and allow us to see *their* tears
- God's peace that passes all understanding, His directing of the next step to take, and the encouragement He provides in so many unexpected ways at just the needed time
- our dear hospitable friend who only lives minutes from SMH opened her home to me for the duration

10/23/14 - Day of Rest

Today was a day of rest for Dale and rest/respite for me as well. He was finally able to sleep through the night with a great amount of medical assistance; slept for much of the day as well, waking for meals and OT. He sang along with a lot of songs and interacted with his caregivers. I met with doctors and therapists. Each of us have a threshold of what we can take, and Dale had reached overload yesterday—lack of sleep, no food for twelve hours due to TEE, anesthesia, meds given later than scheduled due to TEE and…his sight is impaired - how frustrating! The goal is to give him rest and get his days and nights straightened out so he can once again move forward in rehab. We'll post when he'll be able to have visitors again but will be guarding his energy and his time very carefully.

Well, *fortuitous* describes my lunch hour. Praise the Lord! I was walking in the nearby Hillview area on this beautiful sunny, breezy day and heard my name called out, then "Aunt Donna!" Our niece Michelle was driving by on her way to help a friend. We had lunch together out in the fresh air. What a treat and good conversation... definitely a God appointment; two minutes one way or the other and we wouldn't have connected. Loved it! Then I went with family to Christy's district volleyball game—a BIG win over significant rival Fort Myers High School! I am blessed to be part of this volleyball family. Dale will be thrilled!

10/24/14 - ...And then There's God

Another rather peaceful day, thankfully. Although Dale slept in short intervals last night, it was without sedatives. He has enjoyed listening to your notes, studying color cards, and listening to his new Guitar Masters playlist. I didn't see any doctors today but talked with a PA around dinner time. I would like to know how things are progressing toward rehab, but, as Christy reminded me, they are giving him time to adjust and regulate... T-I-M-E. *So, I wait...not the least bit in charge...and learn the balance of my work and my rest.*

When our rabbi friend visited the other day, his wife shared one of his recent phrases with me "*....and then there's GOD.*" I asked him what he had to share with us; here's my paraphrase: "Tell Dale in his confusion of brain damage, go to GOD, rest in Him. Let doctors work on physical; work hard to apply yourself in rehab. After that, your job is to rest in the Lord when you are not working. *Do your part, let medical staff do their part... and then there's GOD.*"

My work, being at one with Dale, is to discern, encourage, and be his advocate. After that, my job also is to rest in the Lord. Like many of us, I'm not used to having much time for rest, so in this time I must practice the presence of God by "quieting the left-brain chatter," resting, trusting and listening. I'm learning...

"In quietness and in confidence will be your strength"   Isaiah 30:15

"Trust in The Lord with all your heart and lean not unto your own understanding. In all your ways acknowledge Him and He will direct your paths"   Proverbs 3:5-6

"You will keep in perfect peace him whose mind is steadfast, because he trusts in You. Trust in the Lord forever, for the Lord, the Lord, is the Rock eternal."   Isaiah 26: 3-4

"Your ears shall hear a word behind you, saying, 'This is the way, walk in it,' whenever you turn to the right hand or whenever you turn to the left."   Isaiah 30:21

10/25/14 - Fresh Air!!

Dale napped a couple of hours this morning after having only about three total hours overnight; he was peaceable most of the time. David visited today while I went to get a massage at Melodie's and then to Patti's for brunch. It is good for me to have breaks. (I was told by one of the patient safety attendants that **suggestions for caregivers are to have one hour off for every three hours on and one day off every three days on**. It makes sense to take care of yourself so you can be healthy to take care of others.)

Doctor came today and agreed that although Dale still has a one-on-one attendant, together the two of us could take him out of the unit today so we went to the atrium for some fresh air and a view of the city. Also, Patti and Bill visited for a while, bringing Dale another great smoothie. He's still overstimulated by things quite easily; his brain is already working hard to recover. Visits will continue to be very limited and dependent on his activities, rest, and energy levels. The request to move him to CRU (rehab) is waiting for an evaluation to be done by their personnel, hopefully on Monday... and then, of course, approval by insurance.

It makes sense to take care of yourself so you can be healthy to take care of others

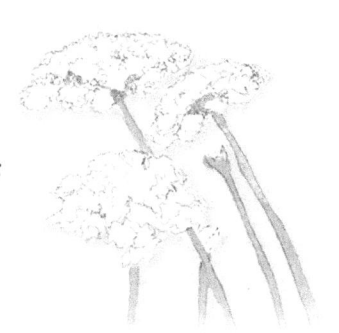

I'm learning so much and am grateful for those who share their knowledge with me be it medical, practical, or spiritual. Many of you will smile to know that I'm having to quiet myself (yes, including the volume of my voice) to help Dale maintain the balance he needs. This means I can't just plow forward with all my "good ideas" but need to carefully listen to the Holy Spirit to direct every step I take—my actions, words, even my thoughts (which is a good thing). My heart might be right and my motivation good, but I don't have the knowledge that I need to know how to help him in this situation. (Encouragement from a dear friend who has experience with TBI reminded me that *"NO ONE has the needed knowledge when brain trauma touches a relationship. That you have laid hold of understanding so quickly and thoroughly is actually your guarantee of greatest success. You've chosen to be perceptive, receptive, and responsive. 'A woman of strengths is a crown for her*

husband.'" -Proverbs 12:4 So, I'm learning to walk circumspectly and more slowly, and appreciate your prayers for me, too.

10/26/14 - Day of Rest

Friends and loved ones,
You have lifted us so much with your posts and prayers. I especially appreciate turning to your notes and knowing I'll always find that someone has heard directly what they need to share with me. You are a part of our journey, and it's precious to us. Dale listens carefully to your messages when he can, usually engaging us in memories as he has energy. He's very quiet as I read to him and focuses on absorbing what you've written.

Today was a day of rest. After learning that Dale had another night of choppy sleep, I **insisted** that the nurse get an answer today from the doctor re: a sedative that will work with Dale's present meds. He rested over an hour after I arrived and ate breakfast by himself for the first time since last Sunday. The nurse practitioner came in and had some good advice including keeping the lights down for less stimulation. I requested a recliner instead of the rocker so that if he falls asleep, he can stay there, and she got it for us right away. We kept everything low key today, had some chair massage and lots of quiet, although we walked some. We got an answer from the doctor late in the afternoon and Dale will have a sedative tonight; I am most grateful for the response. Dale has been getting dissatisfied toward the end of the day (no surprise and actually a *good* sign that he cares), and, as my presence seems to add to his dissatisfaction and he responds better to the staff, I head home. That's the hardest part of my day, leaving him; yet, he does seem to acknowledge that as a step in our routine now and that in itself is a blessing.

Today I'm especially thankful for:
    -my family in Sarasota who are adjusting their lives to help

-David's family being nearby and our grandsons who bring the 'normal' back into view as we play games and share life
-phone calls when I have the time and energy to talk - I do love hearing your voices even for a few minutes
-Christy's daily Snapchats - smiles and ten second snaps of life continuing...
-the beauty of driving down Manasota Key - canopied roads and beach views so close I could see dolphins from my car!

10/27/14 The Healing Power of Sleep

Today was a good day. Dale got five hours sleep last night and then another 2½ hours before I arrived at 10:00 a.m. – yay!

The difference was immense, and his attendant noted for me all the various differences he saw in Dale from three days ago: conversant, took direction well, fed himself, found his own socks, put on his clothes, mouth worked better for drinking, could see better and turned his head as needed to locate things. His nurse had told me that when he walked around this morning he was doing 'high knees;' later today, he did leg lifts on his bed and when we went into the courtyard, he did body weight squats and one leg step-ups on a garden bench! What a difference rest makes in the body! We have a wonderful young man as Dale's safety attendant. They have a great connection, and he is truly a blessing to us both.

Most of us recognize that we function better with rest, but this change is a testimony to the way our bodies were created to need and utilize rest for our health and well-being. We continue to keep the room subdued between activities today just to be able to have rest. So grateful for this progress; still waiting to hear about moving to rehab but have started much on our own. Thank you for your encouragement and prayers.

Today's firsts (in addition to doing exercises):
- went outside in the courtyard to walk and work with letters
- drank a few sips of ginger ale with no coughing
- engaged in lengthy conversation with understanding
- wanted to wear his Coach Hutch wristband
- asked about his watch
- had FaceTime with Christy because he had questions about volleyball playoffs. She showed him the girls warming up for practice in the gym. He later got up from a short nap insistent that he had to go to practice!
- asked for giant dominoes that he had used when at rehab
- was more peaceful when I left even though he was sad

10/28/14 Rest Needed - Again

I'm asking for prayer and wisdom regarding Dale's sleep. After a good day yesterday, he had no sleep *at all* last night. It's 8:00 a.m. and I'm heading down to hopefully be able to meet with doctors but need wisdom and prayer that they will find the answer to help him rest.

Doing my part... and only my part! After hearing that Dale basically got no sleep last night, I felt *my role today was to speak up for his obvious needs, to ask questions and get answers.*

Interestingly, Dale was responding to staff better than to me most of the day so, although I was usually within earshot, I had time to formulate questions for each individual with whom I expected to meet. I believe God gave us the gift of all of today's personal caregivers and was quite overwhelmed to find that his day nurse was the daughter of one of Dale's coaching friends! An immediate bright spot to remind me "... *and then there's God.*"

I reviewed info on Dale's medications/schedule over the past three weeks to clarify what I saw happening. In addition, I got some insight from a dear family friend that gave me further direction. By the end of the morning, Dale had gotten several hours sleep, eaten breakfast and lunch by himself and this afternoon we did get time outside in the courtyard. By the end of my afternoon's meetings:
-everyone was on board that sleep is Dale's #1 priority,
-neuro was signed back on his case and scheduled an EEG for morning to rule out any further stroke activity,
-psych adjusted his meds and put him on the sedative that had previously helped him get a full night's sleep and would follow up at 11:00 p.m. to check effectiveness,
-and written instructions were posted in his room for all shifts of caregivers to see.

That was my part; I left at 5:30 p.m. to let the medical staff do their parts in capably taking care of Dale.

... and then there's God. I am so grateful for His direction and peace, for sending wisdom through just the right person at the right time and blessings when we need a lift. Thank you for doing your part in prayer, encouragement, advice, and TLC.

10/29/14 Praise God!

Dale slept through the night! Hallelujah! Just wanted you all to know. We are expecting a good day.

From a friend:
"There is an interesting article in November's *Prevention* Magazine that I read last night regarding relatively new research that indicates that meditation is actually sleep's most natural partner and in fact mirrors the initial non-REM

phase of sleep which appears to be the most critical phase for basic brain restoration (the article is speaking about a healthy individual). Apparently both meditation and this first stage of sleep synchronize the firing of the brain neurons that fire intermittently in different parts of the brain during typical waking hours. Their thought is that the synchronization may reset neurons and reduce information overload in the brain. The meditation also improves sleep and allows the brain to more effectively rid itself of cellular "trash." If he could manage it, perhaps after doing rehab work, some simple guided meditation could help to "reboot his brain" a few times a day and perhaps to even help him sleep better at night."

And I say THANK YOU! Any and all helpful information is carefully considered.

Looking for the next step. Can you help?
Friends, before I write my update tonight, my family wants you to know our need and contact us personally or through Caring Bridge if you have any resources as we look for the next rehab for Dale. It's a more complex and unique situation than we initially thought and falls outside the range of Acute Rehab or Skilled Nursing Facilities. Specifically, we are looking for:
- inpatient care in the Naples area so I could live with Christy or in the Sarasota area where I have daily family support
- intensive rehab for speech, cognitive, visual, and occupational therapies
- individualized program for traumatic brain injury and neurobehavioral rehab. Thank you for your help.

As I posted earlier, Dale slept through the night...and on through much of the day until 3:00 p.m., getting up very groggy only to use the bathroom. So actually, I had a day of respite for the most part, arriving late morning to meet with caregivers and the rep from a rehab center we're considering... even though it's not near family. They rescheduled SLP and his EEG for tomorrow morning; sleep specialist doctor visited and said to **let him sleep**! I actually left for home around 1:30 p.m. since Dale was still sleeping soundly, leaving him good hands.

Updates later today were that he awoke around 3:00 p.m. and stayed awake, ate dinner, and took night meds on schedule per sleep doctor.

I was able to go with David and Caleb to Christy's regional volleyball quarterfinals game which they won handily.

I'm sure you have noted that I write most of these posts late at night; it is a good recap for me as well as an update for you, and therapeutic as well. Gives me the opportunity to see an overview, assess the needs, and count the blessings. God is in control; all of this is far more than I know and understand. I'm leaning, learning, and following.

"Who is this coming up from the wilderness, Leaning upon her beloved?" -Song of Solomon 8:5 *This describes ME; I am coming up from the wilderness; God is my beloved and is holding me up.* He is faithful and I want to be found faithful as well as I humbly pour out our needs and receive so much from others—care, wisdom, direction, love, gifts, shelter, food, and encouragement. **Thank you**. On a light note, my sister Patti noted today (with grace for the situation) that I've lost the perfection of my "inner editor" in these late hours:) - hah! Over the years, many of you have relied on me for proofreading and now, in the weariness, emotion, and late hours, I fall short, and you get to read my skips and misspellings. Hopefully, I still make sense! *"Forgiven and free"* as my sister Nancy says. If I am again available to proofread for any of you, rest assured it will not be at this late hour! Sweet sleep to us all.

10/30/14 Hospital Life

After a good seven hours of sleep, breakfast, and a morning nap, Dale was ready to DO something and expected me to help him get on with it! It was bittersweet and good to see his desire for activity, even rehab, but sad that there's not much for him to do that's satisfying. Impaired vision affects so many things, even TV, and the inability to converse frustrates him with visiting and often moves him into overstimulation. 'Boring' was never a word that we used in our home or allowed our kids to use, but that's what Dale's hours have been at times.

Conversely, he had many new tests today including one with an IV, plus two labs to check out his coronary artery. He had an EKG and the resting portion of a stress test; will have the remainder of it in the morning. So, boring didn't describe many of his hours after all as he was poked and prodded and wheeled from place to place! He also had a Speech Therapy session in between and did great! OT came by but couldn't get fit in so will come back tomorrow.

Mid-morning, Dale had complained of chest pain and, after further questioning, his nurse called to have cardiac check him out; thus, the tests. Nothing showed up on EKG; labs showed slight troponin elevation. We haven't gotten other results yet. Again, this evening, he complained of chest pains and leg pains so the response team was called and he had more tests. BP is good, he seems to be fine; he is resting well and took night meds. I'll come early in the morning to give him info as he goes to the stress test. However, today was a taste of hospital life that made him *ready to leave* and he did his best to express this to me and his wonderful nurse. He rightfully expects me to be his ally yet doesn't perceive that I always am, nor does he know the big picture and all that is working on his behalf. He vocalized and emoted to me for quite a while, then I asked if I could talk and told him my frustrations as well and a basic plan for progress. That only helped momentarily. He truly seems best when he's focused on an aspect of rehab; and the goal is to get him stabilized and locate a rehab facility that will meet the complex needs he has. So, I go in his room when I can be a help to him, and I leave for the waiting room when his dissatisfaction gets stirred up and he listens better to others.

Today's blessings:
-a good night's sleep for Dale
-Dale's wonderful nurse, the daughter of a coaching friend
-Dale's main attendant who has connected so well with him
-beautiful weather and a refreshing time in the courtyard
-delicious, healthy lunch and an hour of retreat at Patti's
-closed doors - a 'no' is an answer to prayer, too; we only need one open door
-wisdom and insights from our research friend
-dinner waiting when I got to my friend's house... and she didn't even have to cook it!

10/31/14 Four Weeks Out

Dale slept well last night and was awakened to have his stress test early this morning. After that, he napped until 11:30 a.m. He has been awake since that time and had an EEG this afternoon. I hope to have the results of those tests tonight or tomorrow morning, but actually consider no news to be good news since a report would require immediate attention.

Dale had a session this afternoon with the speech therapist, and she upgraded his food to mechanical soft. He also listened to much of SportCenter™ and reacted to a number of comments/opinions.

I spent several hours today talking with administrators of several rehab facilities; insurance has preapproved a rehab place in Tampa. Christy, David, and I will meet Dale's sister Kim there tomorrow for a tour before our final decision, but it does sound like they have what he needs. And gratefully Kim and Kevin are preparing for me to stay with them just 30 minutes away!

"And we know that all things work together for good to those who love God, to those who are the called according to His purpose"
Romans 8:28

Tonight will be four weeks since Dale's stroke. Although he has made great gains, especially with his recovery of the use of his right side, he still has a lot of work ahead of him. Restoration is in progress, in some way every day; today, we noticed changes in his speech as his mouth and tongue restoration has continued to improve.

"God is our Refuge and God is our Strength, a very present Help in trouble. Therefore, I shall not fear, though the earth be removed and though the mountains will tumble into the midst of the sea."
Psalm 46:1-2

11/1/14 Gators 38 Dawgs 20… and Visual Clarity

Last night, after three years without a win over Georgia, Dale's Florida Gators looked great in their 38-20 win over the Dawgs; and… after four weeks without being able to see or concentrate on the TV, Dale was victorious both in watching and engaging in the entire game, including commercials! In addition, they showed a clip from his own 1970 team's FL/GA game, and **he was in it!!** He even got the quiz question right knowing the two coaches were Doug Dickey and Vince Dooley! (For any of you who don't know, Dale played offensive guard for the Gators from 1968 -1971 along with teammates John Reaves and Carlos Alvarez who were mentioned in the TV clip.) ***Very exciting!***

Recap: Yesterday, when I arrived at 7:45 a.m., Dale had slept well, had already done his "workout" of pushups, sit-ups, and wall squats—all on his own accord. After making plans with his very capable attendant for the next few hours, I left to drive with Christy and David for Tampa rehab facility tour. Kim and Kevin met us there and we spent the next 1½ hours learning of their programs, seeing the fine facility firsthand, and asking all our questions. We are ready to move forward with Dale's admission there, which is only pending a personal evaluation from their staff which should take place by Monday. So, over the next few days we'll be making preparation for another big adjustment, and you can be praying for us in that.

Christy and David then had a good visit with their dad. It actually turned quite emotional when they told him of the plan to move to rehab; unpleasant memories came to the surface of other transitions in the past month. They were able to encourage him with descriptions and pictures as well as our promise to be there with him through this change. We may not know the details of his reactions and fears until he can clearly describe them to us, but there are obviously tender moments especially from the early post-stroke days with such poor vision and little understanding. Please pray for his healing of those memories and peace in his heart as we go forward.

After a shave and a shower, Dale was ready to watch the FL/GA game with me and his Gator-loving attendant. He interacted about plays, had much to express about players and what he saw, and laughed at commercials when they were funny. **You need to know that _until 2 days_ ago he couldn't see the TV well enough to follow nor did he have the attention span to even "watch" SportCenter™.** Having received good rest for five nights now and having day medications out of his system has made a HUGE difference in his clarity and understanding. It has also moved him to look forward to getting out of the hospital, although those conversations can be quite trying for everyone.

Dale is still challenged by chronological order, complex thinking, and following more than one-step directions. However, it is familiar and comforting to our family to see him go into "automatic pilot" when he brushes teeth, puts on shirts/socks/shoes in the same way he always has. He misses family, friends, home, and familiar places; it's been a month with more to come. David, Steph, and grandsons are coming Sunday afternoon; a dear coaching friend will visit today; there is football on TV and sunshine outside. Much to look forward to and we thank you for sharing in this journey.

11/2/14 A Cheerful Heart is Good Medicine

Lots of love and laughter - a wonderful day! *"A cheerful heart is good medicine"*   *Proverbs 17:22*

Another good night's sleep for both of us; so grateful that Dale is now having regular days and nights. I arrived around 9:00 a.m. as Dale was finishing breakfast and ready to shower. At 10:00 a.m., we had a wonderful and lengthy visit with his dear friend with whom he both coached and taught; what a precious time! They talked about so many things and caught up on family; it was a time to treasure and was only interrupted for an OT session. Lots of joking, memories, and laughter; Dale was quite tired by the time the visit was over and rested for about thirty minutes before lunch but didn't sleep. It is good to see that he has the energy to make it through the day. OT was very helpful. Dale is doing very well with identifying items and copying them; visual impairment does affect this in many ways, but we can still measure progress. Dale was thoroughly engaged, and the therapist gave us some specific things to work on.

David, Steph, and the boys visited for nearly two hours; we went out in the courtyard, threw a football, walked and talked in the fresh air, then sat in the bright and cheerful lobby and shared life. The boys shared their grades, endeavors, sports plans, and piano updates; Dale shared his new words and sounds. His normal sense of humor quickly had us all laughing! After we went back to Dale's room, we laughed aloud at the jokes that McKinleys have been faithful to send. When the family left, Dale was ready to follow, and we had a "moment" that sometimes comes upon us when his understanding hasn't quite caught up with the reality of our circumstances.

Patti and Bill came by with a healthy shake which Dale loves. Bill reported on his century bike ride of 100 miles today. He dedicated it to Dale/Coach Hutch, wore his wristband, and purposely prayed for Dale when his ride became an effort. Very interesting to note that this year's CycleFest colors were orange and blue, so Bill was decked out in Gator colors as he rode for Dale! We had a great visit walking together in the bright and cheerful lobby and courtyard.

Many times today, we had opportunity to review the steps with Dale re: his upcoming transition, the various things that have to happen and the order in which they'll happen, pictures of where we expect to go, discussion of cities and surroundings and the family that will be with him, nearby, and visiting. Since he doesn't have a good concept of time or order, his expectations still surface according to what he wants to happen, and we have to review it all again. I am/we are glad that he wants to move forward and isn't satisfied sitting around; that's very healthy, but it is sad when he realizes it's not happening *now*, that I have to go home, and he has to stay. *It is a very hard time of my day.*

So thankful for:
- kind and competent nursing staff
- caring patient safety attendants who interact so well with Dale and our family/friends
- laughter and smiles
- sunshine even on a cold Florida day
- the Gator football victory over Georgia
- Dale's high school friend sending us a pic that took us down memory lane
- friends from all stages of our life
- Dale being able to watch football on TV when I left tonight
- David and Stephanie raising their children to love family and enjoy interacting with adults
- time to go home, rest and refresh, and pack up for the next phase of this journey
- sweet sleep

11/3/14 A Good Day

A good day...after a good night's sleep...so there's much for which we are thankful:
- doctors who care, listen, and explain
- medical staff who take a personal interest in their patients and families
- beautiful courtyard/cheerful lobby we can enjoy with others
- plans for Dale to move to a NeuroRehab facility this week
- friends that drove up from Englewood to visit
- Patti and the healthy shakes she's made for Dale
- Dale's progress in communicating, eating real food (soft) and drinking water
- Dale's interest in working on relearning numbers and letters
- all our friends and family who are doing their part - research, encouragement, notes, calls, visits, prayer - often regarding things we wouldn't have thought of or known about

God is good; our trust is in Him as He leads us step by step. Please continue to pray for Dale's continued recovery and the transition to the next phase of his restoration. We are blessed and you are part of the blessing, so we pray God's blessing on you and yours today.

"Rejoice in the Lord always. I will say it again: Rejoice! Let your gentleness be evident to all. The Lord is near. **Do not be anxious about anything, but in everything, by prayer and petition, with thanksgiving, present your requests to God. And the peace of God, which transcends all understanding, will guard your hearts and your minds in Christ Jesus.**

Finally, brothers, whatever is true, whatever is noble, whatever is right, whatever is pure, whatever is lovely, whatever is admirable--if anything is excellent or praiseworthy—think about such things."
Philippians 4:4-8

Chapter Three

NEUROREHAB

11/4/14 The Next Step

Dale's admission to NeuroRehab Services Florida (NSF) in Tampa was confirmed late this afternoon and we are thrilled. It looks like discharge and transport will take place in two days, early Thursday. After five family members visited NSF this past Saturday, we were all confident that this is the place for Dale's next step in rehab and are grateful that all has worked together to make that a reality. The patient's room is very much like a hotel, the gathering rooms are bright and welcoming, and the staff and program are well-suited to meet Dale's complex neuro/cognitive/communication needs along with OT and daily living restoration. In addition to their OT/PT gym, there are two porches, an outdoor walking area with a pond, and planned local field trips—MOSI, mall, swimming pool, etc.

Although we'll be farther from immediate family, I will be staying with Dale's sister and brother-in-law about thirty minutes from the rehab. We have a few friends in the Tampa area and encourage our friends from elsewhere to let us know when you want to visit while when traveling to nearby USF, MOSI, or Busch Gardens. Once we know Dale's schedule, we can set up times to visit.

Dale had a good day again, thankfully, with visits from Patti and our pastor. The visits were most welcome. Dale's doctor had changed night meds and came in today to fine tune those as he works toward solid hours of rest during the night. Dale passed his swallow test today for thin liquids and can now use a straw as well. He's ready to go and get on with the rehab. In the meantime, we've got puzzles and flashcards, numbers and letters, drawing, and large dominoes to work with. In addition, our nephew Michael suggested a Powerball gyro hand exerciser so we were able to get one today and will begin utilizing it for hand strength and dexterity; very cool.

Tomorrow will be a day to prepare for the move, finalize transportation, and say goodbye to those who have cared so well for us in the past 2½ weeks. We appreciate your prayers as we transition and settle into a new place, new facility, and. new routine. And Dale's sleep is still a matter for prayer.

11/5/14 Where He Leads

Dale will be discharged in the morning, and we'll leave for Tampa. Today was a wonderful day spent with our caregivers at the hospital with many words of encouragement, well-wishes, handshakes, and hugs after sixteen days together through emotion and victory.

Dale made significant mental progress today: the wooden numbers puzzle that he labored over yesterday and partially completed before exhausting himself was completed by him today within five minutes! Exponential change! Hallelujah! I watched in amazement.

This morning as I packed my car at home for an unknown period of time, I was thankful for the twenty-five years that I've worked daily out of my car and traveled often enough to learn to pack and plan ahead as much as possible. But here I stood, not knowing when I'll be home again or how long we'll be in Tampa or what we'll face on a daily basis. I was reminded of my reflections of several years ago, when after moving twice in two years, we faced the possibility of another move. I was resistant to even think about it, but God showed me His truth about His people following Him, both journeying and camping at His direction (Numbers 9:15-23). So, as we move again, going through the doors that have opened before us, I share with you my journal reflections formerly recorded in February 2011:

"We've been "empty-nesters" for many years as our children moved on, yet in the literal sense, we've rarely had an empty nest. As we've yielded our home to God, He has continually filled it with His people as He chose in His time. I am a nester, HOME-maker, the maker of a HOME - settle in, fluff things up, take care of the nest and those in it, push them out when they're ready, make a new nest when the old one is damaged, or we "migrate". I would be happy to have HOME in one place all of my life, going out as needed but returning HOME, any the Father brings to us.

*This nesting satisfies both my spirit and my flesh, yet primarily I am not a nester, but a God-follower - wherever He leads in the spiritual or the physical. I've gone places I never expected or even wanted to go - spiritually and physically, and, in sharing our home with others, we've been tested in ways we never would have chosen, yet His grace is sufficient (you think??) and we are sharpened by one another (*Proverbs 27:17 NIV*). In my weakness (emotional, self-centered, from past hurts/traumas, whatever), He is made strong. The Amplified Bible expounds on this, "But He (the Lord) said to me, My grace (My favor and lovingkindness and mercy) is enough for you; for My strength and power are made perfect (fulfilled and completed) and show themselves." 2 Corinthians 12:9*

My desire is that I glorify God - I cannot determine how that will happen; I must trust His leading. "'For My thoughts are not your thoughts, nor are your ways My ways,' says the Lord. 'For as the heavens are higher than the earth, so are My ways higher than your ways, and My thoughts than your thoughts.'" Isaiah 55:8-9 NKJV

Humbling, isn't it? I can't even choose how to glorify Him...and yet, I choose to obey implicitly and immediately, trusting Him wholly. He is faithful, worthy; He is love itself. I do choose to glorify Him, to follow Him where He leads.

Nesting? Following God? As believers we have nomadic heritage even from before our father Abraham to the children of the Exodus who followed the pillar of cloud and fire. Our innate desire is to hear His voice and follow Him. Let us encourage one another to readily to move out at His direction, to pick up our tent (spiritual or physical), taking only what is essential, leaving the rest behind. Hanging onto ways or things of the past will only hold us back from all He has for us. We do well to read and learn from Old Testament stories of God's people in bondage in Egypt, delivered from that bondage, yet wandering in the wilderness because of their stubbornness. Isaiah 43 tells of God's protection, His love, <u>His</u> plan for His people - not our plan. "Do not remember the former things, nor consider the things of old. Behold, I will do a new thing, now it shall spring forth; shall you not know it? I will even make a road in the wilderness and rivers in the desert."   Isaiah 43: 18-19 NKJV

Following hard after Him? There is no better way!"

11/6-7/14 Arriving at Tampa Rehab

Thursday was quite the day and not without a few snags, just enough to remind me I'm not in control and to listen for direction. Dale actually slept soundly all night (unlike me) and I had to wake him when I arrived at 7:30 a.m.! Hallelujah! He was ready for the day. Melodie arrived to help us pass the time, giving us both chair massages—a wonderful blessing. Patti and our attendant friend helped with the drive and transition to NeuroRehab Services Florida (NSF) near USF in Tampa.

Once there, Dale was very pleased with accommodations and personnel and settled well. The only exception was when he questioned a timeline and realized he would not be leaving after the weekend. We just can't know what's in his mind and, no matter how we try to communicate clearly and cover all the bases, he is not yet able to tell us what he's thinking. God provided a revelation of the time Dale and I lived under separate roofs as he transitioned to the head football coach position in Sebring, nearly two months of only weekends together. I was able to remind him that we weathered that just fine, even in different towns, and that now we'll be seeing each other nearly every day. Today we shared that with the NSF staff so they can continue to encourage us as time goes on. Right now, we don't know the timeline, but weekly goals will be set, and Dale has already been diligent in working hard to recover.

We continue to be encouraged and Dale is social with his new team and fellow patients; so am I. In addition to practicing homework with the staff, he is playing bingo and cards in the capacity he can and watching TV with his attendant. This is a small group facility, and we actually see quite a ministry for us to those here, especially those with few visitors. I plan to be there every day except for respite days; admin has already issued me a family/volunteer picture ID, is setting me up for official volunteer certification, and included me in the noon meal. I have volunteered to proofread/edit for them and to cook some for Thanksgiving and special occasions. God's grace is abundant as we open our hearts to those with whom He has placed us. In fact, today we were greatly blessed to connect with Englewood friends who will be within a mile or so at Moffitt over the next few weeks as he has surgery. We all agree that God is giving us this opportunity to encourage and strengthen one another during their time here in Tampa. What a mighty God we serve! His plans are SO far above ours; higher than the heavens are above the earth.

My sister-in-law told me she watched Caring Bridge all day today to see when I'd post; I can only say that I'll do this as I can and encourage you to have post notifications sent to you if you're interested. I was exhausted last night and didn't leave NSF until around 11:00 p.m. after I'd met the night shift staff. That was not my plan, but I was then able to sleep well all night and so was Dale. Thank you, Lord.

Kim and Kevin have a wonderful place for me and their dogs are already adjusting to me invading *their* space. Kim reminded that *she is a caregiver* and will be taking care of me. I am most grateful.

Dale can have visitors; weekends are especially good. However, as he finishes evaluation and is in an established rehab routine, I'll still be guarding his energy and rest. Please contact me by email or phone/text if you are planning to visit. We'd love to see you!

On another note, Dale's dear friend from back in high school has set up a GoFundMe account for us to offset expenses not covered by insurance. Friends are priceless.

11/9/14 "Family"

Dale and I have always had an open home since we were married. That openness had been modeled to me from my parents who first had my maternal grandparents live with them. One Christmas season when I was in elementary school, a girl named Pam from an orphanage came and stayed with us for the holidays. After I left for college, in addition to my grandparents, several families and many individuals lived in Mom and Dad's home and were welcomed as family, staying as long as needed.

Dale and I hosted our own first "family addition" in 1976 when Christy was an infant. Over the years, we've had dozens of wonderful individuals and even two entire families live with us. It has been a rich heritage and one that our children now share with us.

Here at NSF, we are joining a new family and are learning our roles. Dale, as "Coach," has already started an arcade basketball tournament and joined the group for workouts at the nearby gym. I'll be working with the Activities Director so I can cook on the weekends; patients will choose healthy foods, plan menus, and make grocery lists. One of our new friends is from Poland; I'll be bringing my grandmother's Polish cookbook and a Polish newspaper that was my dad's. Another new friend is originally from Guatemala; one is from NC and the other from FL. Not many families visit - the FL parents come briefly every two weeks and the NC wife as they can work it out, so Dale and I are providing much of the family atmosphere and, of course, our own family members will be involved as they visit here.

Please pray for these precious new friends as they, too, have had their lives turned upside down and are working hard to recover. And pray for us to be a blessing right where we are with Kim and Kevin's family and the staff here as well as with the other patients. Other prayer requests:
- continued settling in for Dale
- his improved understanding of his situation
- ways to increase the healthy food options
- workout options for me
- an opportunity for me to go home/Englewood for a few days

11/11/2014 Visitors

Over the weekend we welcomed visits from family, a real pleasure since Dale hasn't settled into routine yet and has had much down time. Kim came with me for most of Saturday and Kevin joined us mid-afternoon. On Sunday Christy, David, and Matthew came for much of the afternoon. We are both lifted by visits and appreciate the effort to make the trip and work with the communication. It is rewarding to see Dale respond to everyone and to hear him tell of his pleasure with NSF and the staff, to show everyone what he's doing and learning, and to share the beauties of the property. Weather permitting, we can take everyone outside to the lake and boardwalk where there are opportunities to enjoy nature such as ducks, fish, ibis, and even a couple of Malibu wood storks.

On Saturday, we were totally surprised to meet a fellow Gator football letterman! Being a game day, Dale had on his Gator gear and a gentleman approached him on the boardwalk and introduced himself by saying that he, too, played football for UF in 1944! Wow! They shared details—both were O-line, nearly the same playing size and our new friend pulled out his F Club Letterwinner's card, the present one as well as the original! His wife is getting nursing care right now and their daughter is visiting; their home is actually a condo across the street. Small world... what a pleasure!

Dale still struggles with timelines, grasping the whole picture, and, consequently, impatience. These are all products of the left-brain trauma and continue to arise from time to time. Fortunately, he will bring these up and actually "vents" quite a lot to me, as he should. We got family counseling on Saturday so he could hear from an expert re: more details and expectations. This was good for all of us, Kim and Kevin expressed their appreciation of her expertise and manner in which she spoke with Dale. On Sunday, Dale was able to express his feelings to both Christy and David; we realized he often gets facts mixed up and these talk times give us opportunity to reinforce the truth. So grateful that Dale trusts both staff and family.

We are ready for visitors as long as we know ahead of time and can guard Dale's energy and time. Friends from Englewood came over Monday afternoon while in town for a medical visit at Moffitt. It was so good to share a time of catching up and encouraging one another. I will be staying together with her at her hotel for a week after his upcoming surgery, so this was great preparation and confirmed that decision. This friend is a barber and brought his barber tools, gave Dale a haircut and trimmed his beard. It was just as if he set up shop and Dale walked in! It was good interaction for them both! I wish I had taken a picture, but the memory of it will linger for all of us.

Dale is doing well at NSF and had a good day today, yet fears surface with emotion and we are facing them head on, now with the help of an on-staff counselor who is available to us and our families. We praise God for those who are ministering to us in this place, many of whom have strong relationships with our Father. We can rest in His care for us and the hands that provide it. Dale has now progressed to not needing a nighttime one-on-one attendant, with staff now checking on him every fifteen minutes during the night... another step forward.

S-T-R-O-K-E

Since our lives so obviously turned upside down within a moment at 10:00 p.m., October 3rd, we have continuously been learning about stroke and brain injury, yet also know there is so much more to learn. Although Dale and I knew some signs of stroke, neither of us knew about killer headaches such as the one Dale had on the mid-afternoon of October 3rd.

We and our family were marginally aware of several of the stroke warning signs but have learned that in the U.S. a stroke occurs nearly every minute, is one of the leading causes of death, and the annual cost of stroke is in the billions of dollars. Unfortunately, most people don't know that stroke can strike anyone, anytime, anywhere. So, I'm encouraging everyone to get a better understanding, even looking at current info and statistics.

STROKE is a medical emergency. Call 9-1-1

Here are a couple of acronyms that can help us all to recognize stroke and get help FAST:

Warning Signs Of Stroke

S = SPEECH, or any problems with talking
T = TINGLING, or any numbness in the body
R = REMEMBER, or any problems with memory
O = OFF BALANCE, problems with coordination
K = KILLER HEADACHE
E = EYES, or any problems with vision

>F = FACE droops
>A = ARM weakness, can't raise
>S = SPEECH difficulty, slurring
>T - TIME to call **9-1-1**

11/12/14 Caregivers...

"In everything, do to others what you would have them do to you."

Dale is in a great place, and I am learning that as we adjust, I must retreat and allow/encourage him to struggle through communication with those who are caring for him so he can trust them and be restored into self-governance, not relying on me as his interpreter. He is working hard; today, his focus was to say my name. I told him yesterday that God understands him when he talks to Him no matter how he sounds, but if he wants to ask about me when I'm not there, he needs to be able to say my name. So today, he had a goal and met it—to say my name correctly... over and over and over. If I have the story straight, he took my picture out of the frame on his dresser and brought it to speech therapy. So, they worked on my name (among many other things) and all day he would hold up my picture to others or to me so we could speak "Donna" to him, and he would listen carefully and repeat it correctly. I love it; especially because I see how hard he is working and because he can see success!

> *"In everything, do to others what you would have them do to you."*

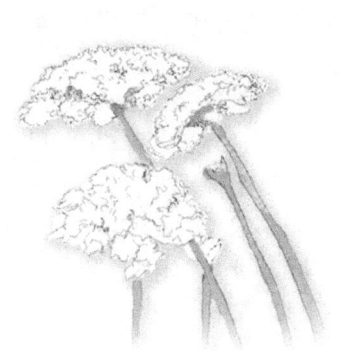

I am so thankful for caregivers. For the past six weeks, we have been receiving care—urgent care, medical care, pastoral care, personal care, food, housing, laundry, prayer, research and gathering resources, phone calls, cards, stories, and jokes—all working together to meet our needs. Whether it's your job, your duty, your ministry, your gifting or talent, to give of yourself with lovingkindness and selflessness is to be a blessing to others. We've been blessed and continue to be blessed as we receive care. Right now, as I live in Kim and Kevin's home, they have opened their house, rearranged furniture, disrupted schedules and family pets, made breakfast and dinner, and even washed my clothes. I am blessed and my family has peace regarding my well-being.

Caring for Dale right now, I'm drawing on the life experiences we've had as well as those of others before and around us and absorbing the knowledge of other caregivers from all walks of life, recognizing the balance of overseeing or relinquishing care to others; making decisions or allowing Dale to do so as he can; taking charge or trusting others with his care; being present or taking respite. Dale and I have been mentored in caregiving over decades through many individuals in our families, a rich heritage on both sides. My parents cared for my maternal grandparents; my paternal grandfather cared for his wife until death, then my parents cared for him; my dad cared for mom until she died; my sister Patti and brother Rick cared for them both in various ways as needs surfaced; Dale's grandmother was cared for by her children; his sister Kim along with her family cared for their mom through dementia up until her death; brother-in-law Kevin's parents cared for his grandmother; sister-in-law Melodie's parents cared for her grandmother, then she and Rick and family cared for her mom; brother-in-law Ken's mother was cared for by him and Nancy; sister Carol nursed her husband through brain cancer; daughter-in-law Stephanie's parents help in caring for their families as well. Our families' practices have made it natural for continuing generations to give love and care as needs surface.

This afternoon, we reread many of your notes, encouraging Dale as the strong fighter, hard worker, and disciplined, persevering man of character that you all have known and loved. Thank you. You, too, are caregivers, giving of yourselves to encourage us both. "Be devoted to one another in brotherly love. Honor one another above yourselves...Be joyful in hope, patient in affliction, faithful in prayer. Share with God's people who are in need. Practice hospitality. (Romans 12:10, 12-13)"

As you bless us, we ask:
"The Lord bless you and keep you;
The Lord make His face shine upon you, and be gracious to you;
The Lord lift up His countenance upon you, and give you peace."
Numbers 6:24-26

11/15/2014 Respite & First Day Apart

I'm writing this while riding to Gainesville with Christy and friends, heading to watch football—Gators vs. South Carolina. This is part of my new regimen that combines self-care with Dale's need to trust and rely on his rehab caregivers. This week, I've joined a gym and started working out three times a week with at least two additional cardio days. Dale has started Monday/Wednesday/Friday full therapy days, so I only see him a couple of hours on those days. Today, Kim will visit him for a good part of the day; tomorrow, I'll be there all day and then I have to go home until midday Tuesday so Kim will be visiting him those days.

Quick update on Dale. He's doing GREAT! He has speech therapy every day and is now saying words, sometimes without prompts. He is making great gains and the therapist is thrilled. PT and OT love him, and he's been using the anti- gravity treadmill which is great for his joints. This was a milestone day as Dale and I are apart for an entire day for the first time since the stroke. In fact, by the time I see him tomorrow morning, it will be more than thirty-six hours. I am delighted to report that he had a good day, as did I. Some details:

-he remembered Kim was coming today and,
-before she came, he had told nurses her name several times
-he remembered that I was in Gainesville with Christy
-had Pizza Hut pizza for lunch with his group
-listened to entire Gator game on radio with Kim and followed it all
-did his speech homework several times throughout the day
-had a short but good visit with Christy on her way back through Tampa, and understood why it was a short visit
-asked Christy to repeat several things to him so he could say them himself - that was a first!

There have been many milestones this week. Dale has been released from one-on-one care now that his blood pressure is stabilizing without medication, and he can see better so he doesn't need regular assistance. They taper care off, now checking on him every fifteen minutes, tomorrow every thirty minutes, the next day once an hour like everyone else and that will be maintained. He also knows where to get assistance if he needs help with TV remote, personal care, hygiene, or anything else. He is beginning to understand time better, remembering events from one day to another, and acknowledging that this rehab is for several months, but not for years.

To God be the glory for all this progress. I was reminded today of what I journaled earlier on 10/24: Do your part, let medical staff do their part*... and then there's GOD.*

11/17/14 Moving Forward

Just a quick note to let you know that Dale is continuing to move forward, step by step. Yesterday, Sunday, we spent the day together pretty much by ourselves, outside walking and sitting by the lake, just glad to be in a place where we can enjoy nature. We worked out at the gym and Dale was able to do one set of everything that David had set up for his full body workout with just one short break; our attendant worked out with him, and it was a good start for her! Although the weights are light, he is doing everything correctly and slowly, and doing personal training with a staffer as well! Counting aloud correctly and saying the numbers was greatly improved by the end of the exercises. We also watched "Good Will Hunting," a favorite movie; Dale was totally engaged and readily pointed out upcoming scenes that he loves. It is great to see his vision, memory, and attention being restored.

I have to rejoice that Dale's vision is greatly improved! We were not given false hopes yet knew that any improvement was likely to come in the first two months. Hallelujah, it has! He is recognizing words as large as the title to this journal entry and is interested in what he can glean from the newspaper, asking me to read a few items of particular interest. He can also see pictures on phones. As a gauge for this improvement, at the end of October, he could hardly focus on the TV! We thank God for healing and restoration.

It's still hard for Dale to recognize progress day to day, but therapists, staff and family are reminding him of what they've seen. Today was a full day of therapy, some of which he enjoys more than others. He works hard at it all; his speech therapist is wonderful and so pleased with his progress.

Thank you for your continued prayer and support in every way. Dale now loves to read and even reread your messages and cards.

11/19/14 Another First!

Recently, Dale has made much progress, but it is often hard to describe. In addition, my goal is to share our day-to-day journey, not to be grasping for things to share; sometimes even rehab life is mundane. However, when we have a grateful heart, there always seems to be something for which we are thankful.

Today, Dale got to walk to Planet Smoothie with me; we are thankful. We both enjoy simple pleasures; walking and talking just the two of us, being outside on a beautiful crisp day, sunshine, and exercise. We walked a total of forty-five minutes... and of course, the smoothie topped it off. *This was Dale's first off-site venture.*

It's been several days now that Dale has had hourly check-ins but no one-on-one attendant and has had more time alone or with me or guests, without the constant presence of another person (a regular part of his life since October 3rd). No matter how wonderful a companion might be, we all cherish alone time (consider the mother of young children who even wait outside the bathroom door!). Dale has a continual and growing realization of length of his rehab stay, although there is no specified length of time. We have to remind him that it's not years, not even a year, but months. Many times, this hits him very hard emotionally, exhibited through sadness, heartache, anger, frustration, loss, blame, etc. which rises to the surface and needs to be acknowledged as real and painful. Today as he worked hard to convey his feelings to me and two of the staff, one of them revealed to him that **he could begin have outings with me and family members,** providing of course that these didn't result in arguments or resistant behaviors. She told Dale he could visit our friend at nearby Moffitt once he's out of ICU, that he can go to dinner with Christy and friends this coming Sunday, and that he can even go to his sister's for Thanksgiving! It is very timely for Dale to have these outings offered to him. So, later in the day when I suggested we walk to Planet Smoothie, everyone was on board. (By the way, I usually make him a healthy protein shake but was not able to do that today). AND…since a discussion of Christmas gifts and not being home started today's grieving, this same staffer told Dale that he could have an overnight at home for Christmas! We truly hadn't been thinking that far ahead; I, for one, can hardly consider tomorrow, but God knows what we all need, and Dale now has been given this *gift of anticipation*.

We are blessed by this staff. I could write on and on but know there will be plenty of time for these stories to unfold. Thank God for knowing our every need and thank you for your love and prayers.

11/20/14 Christy's Birthday

Thirty-nine years ago, our precious daughter Christy was born and we celebrate her today. We sent her flowers this morning, called and both sang Happy Birthday to her this afternoon and, Lord willing, will go out to eat with her on coming Sunday. We are blessed with wonderful family relationships, and it has been difficult and emotional for both of us to be in facilities rather than at home.

Emotions often come to the surface for Dale as family comes to mind as well as friends that we are used to seeing. It's particularly hard for Dale when he knows our Englewood grandsons are involved in activities that we would normally attend and support. Right now, they are all wrestling and Dale would be attending those practices and encouraging them in their moves. But even hearing them play piano weekly or watching them play chess at our house was part of our normal life, so that is a very tender spot and you can pray for grace for Dale and a better understanding of the big picture. I'm grateful that he does emote, cry, get very emphatic and even a bit angry about these losses and changes, yet it is difficult for both of us when we have to deal with it. We are blessed with staff that will help us as well and we call on them as God's provision for the moment. But the Lord Himself carries us through and Dale is now at a point in his understanding that we can talk more about relying on God and listening to Him.

We did get to visit our friend today. Both of us went to Moffitt Cancer Center and Dale did very well with the hospital visit, a matter about which family and staff had some concern since Dale had a recent lengthy hospitalization. We had a very nice visit and will hope to see him again in the next week. During this outing, I noticed Dale's progress in the ability to get in the car smoothly, opening and closing the door, and buckling his seatbelt easily; two weeks ago, that was a difficult series of maneuvers.

Your prayers for us continue to be most welcome. Please pray for continued peace and wisdom for nutrition, medication, and overall physical, mental, and spiritual care, and for wisdom and favor regarding medical bills that are coming in.

11/21/14 Dale's Speech

I've had several questions regarding Dale's speech in the past few days. Dale is dealing with both aphasia and apraxia; his speech therapy addresses both. He had two strokes on October 3rd, one dead center in the speech center/Broca's area of the brain. Therefore, the connections that allow speech to happen were damaged and new connections/neural pathways need to be made. Realizing how long it takes for me to explain and how intricate the answer is, I suggest you Google "understanding aphasia" and "aphasia vs. apraxia".

https://www.stroke.org/en/about-stroke/effects-of-stroke/cognitive-and-communication-effects-of-stroke/aphasia-vs-apraxia

Scan here for more information

The brain is changeable; that attribute which happens through learning and practice, development of new habits and neural connections is called neuroplasticity. (Neuroplasticity Made Simple, Phil Parker, PhD)

https://m.youtube.com/watch?v=tJ93qXXYRpU&feature=youtu.be

Scan here for more information

That being said, be assured that Dale's understanding is excellent, and he can engage in conversations involving intricate medical terminology and follow the detailed plays of an entire football game (which many of you cannot, right?). He also is generating conversations about concerns he has, some of which require very complex thinking, and will labor through communication by emphatic speech, gestures, and even some rather funny charades! Although these "conversations" can be tiring for everyone involved, it is VERY encouraging to know that the Dale we know is "still in there" and has much to offer to all of us. He has helped a friend understand her knee pain and get relief, is teaching a female staffer to throw a football correctly at her request, and is helping another start weight-training. In addition, he often prompts me to elaborate on an incident that is appropriate to an ongoing conversation.

The therapy used for Dale's rehab is the PROMPT technique: Prompts for Restructuring Oral Muscular Phonetic Targets

http://promptinstitute.com/index.php?page=what-is-prompt3

Scan here for more information

We have seen great progress in a two-week period and have shared some of that over Caring Bridge. He works five days a week with his speech therapist for a full hour, then has homework to reinforce what he's learned. These exercises can be done hourly for five to ten minutes unless Dale is tired.

Other helpful activities are:
- practicing whistling
- singing Deck the Halls using only la, la, la
- listening to audiobooks
- singing along with music

In addition, family and friends that talk with him can encourage him:
- to say one-word answers;
- to slow down and <u>wait to speak</u>;
- and, when repeating or learning a new word (like the friend's name), we can <u>speak slowly, decreasing our volume</u> as he speaks the word so he can hear himself.

Much learning is taking place, so much that it is hard to list the many daily changes and improvements. Dale can say many words correctly when repeating them and he can also generate some words on his own, saying them correctly.

11/22/2014 Vision Restored!

We're still getting questions about Dale's vision so want to address it today; we firmly believe and see evidence that his eyesight is restored to what it was before the stroke!

Last week, I wrote that Dale's vision is greatly improved. The neurologist here at NSF, explained that homonymous hemianopsia Dale experienced was due to brain swelling from the stroke, impairing visual pathways from the optic chiasm to the visual cortex at the back of the head. *Once swelling subsided, sight was restored.* There was no direct stroke damage to his optic chiasm (had that been the case, vision impairment would likely have been permanent).

When Patti and Bill visited today, they specifically mentioned the great improvement in Dale's sight since they last saw him over two weeks ago; he now can read words, readily finds all his food at meals, has asked for a watch, even fastening the strap. Hallelujah! Restored sight is a huge step forward, significant for Dale's rehab.

In addition to a visit from Patti and Bill (including homemade scones), our dear friend from Lakeland joined us for the day and we all enjoyed time together. Her musical giftings have blessed our entire family for decades now, and it was a pleasure to share encouragement and song together. She also brought Dale a gift bag of much-appreciated healthy snacks which he immediately tested out! What a pleasure to actually have some intimate family time together even in this place of rehab.

Home IS where the heart is, and our hearts are full today.

11/24/2014 You Said if I Belong To You...

On Saturday, when visiting with our Lakeland friend (and Patti and Bill), we had the keyboard out for her. While she played, Patti started singing her favorite song that this friend wrote. As that song finished, I immediately started singing one of her songs that Dale and I have shared countless times throughout the years. However, this time I could hardly get through the first line without tears and sobs... singing these real words to God and hearing His response within the song was emotional; so be it. God can bring release in me (and others) however He sees fit. We made it through the song with our friend playing and filling in words with me. So, I share these words with you now; be encouraged and blessed; He is always with us.

> You said if I belong to You
> Out of me would flow rivers of life.
> I don't mean to make light of it,
> But, Lord, my river sure seems dry.
> But, Lord, my river sure seems dry.
>
> You're using this to be made strong;
> Even when I think I'm right,
> I turn out so wrong.
> I'm to the point I don't know what to do.
> How can I hear clearly from You?
> How can I know it's really You?
> "There will be a sweet peace in your spirit
> Even when things around you seem to fall apart.
> You can rest assured in this, My child:
> I'll never leave your heart."
>
> You said if I belong to You
> Out of me would flow rivers of life.
> So, Lord, even when my river seems dry,
> I know that You will see me through,
> Simply 'cause I belong to You.
> Simply 'cause I belong to You.
> *-Debbie Hester*

11/25/14 Outings!

All is well; Dale continues to get good reports from his therapists. His speech assessment was initially at 24.2 and in two weeks has improved to 36.8; his speech therapist told us that is

REMARKABLE for a two-week period! Thank You, Lord, for a great therapist and Dale's hard work.

Sunday, we both got to go to lunch with Christy and four friends that had been in Gainesville for the weekend. These gals are part of our Naples "family," and we were thrilled to have time with them. Dale did great eating out at the Greek restaurant and had no problem with the food or with making his needs known. He was totally comfortable and engaged in conversation with everyone. They had all read the journal entry on Dale's speech and knew what to expect from talking with Christy as well. Our wellness trainer friend had much to offer when asked about the brain training program she's been studying for two years and is planning to visit us again soon. The other friend's oldest son had brain injury from an accident and this conversation is likely to end up benefitting him as well. I was astounded that these things came up at lunch! I truly had not even considered our time together as being anything other than catching up, but God had other things in mind, and we were totally blessed and encouraged by this visit.

Today, Tuesday, Dale and I got to go off by ourselves for the first time. I needed to make pumpkin pies for the rehab Thanksgiving meal on Wednesday and for Kim's on Thursday. Since I'm staying with our friend at Residence Inn, we have a full kitchen, so we went there for three hours, got the pies made, and Dale got in a workout at the fitness room. We had a few strained moments of conversation and had to discuss patience, slowing down and letting our conversation be the objective without allowing frustration to accelerate. If we're going to have more times with just the two of us, we have to be sure he will be healthy and that we can resolve any issues ourselves if we are to be allowed off site on a regular basis. Dale's understanding is improving so, although concepts still have to be repeated, he is grasping more of the goals and the overall picture as his cognition improves. It was a good time for us and although he was reticent when we drove into the rehab parking lot, he wasn't resistant. There will be time to discuss this with the staff. Tomorrow, we both are being interviewed for the NSF website and are glad to be able to recommend this facility to others. Dale has also been photographed at physical therapy and will have pictures posted on their behalf. It is so interesting to see how we are fitting in and how I am able to give feedback from a patient's family's perspective; it is welcomed and often needed. God is good and is using us right where we are.

11/27/2014 Thanksgiving - We Do Give Thanks!

Praise God from Whom all blessings flow; He is good all the time.

So much for which to be thankful this year:
- God's awesome timing and direction
- first responders and their wise, decisive attention
- opportunity for care at UF Health/Shands Jacksonville
- tPA -amazing clot-busting enzyme that stopped the stroke
- Dale's continual healing
- our children's constant care, feedback, phone calls, visits
- family and friends who stay available 24/7
- supportive, loving extended family
- friendships old and new, some spanning fifty years!
- those loved ones who shelter and feed Donna
- visit with friends at Moffitt (God's timing/blessing for all)
- gifted, caring medical staff and caregivers
- technology that keeps us connected with so many
- Caring Bridge
- humor and laughter
- visits from friends and family near and far
- phone calls, cards, and notes of encouragement
- music and singing
- fresh air and sunshine and the lake at Dale's rehab

-Thanksgiving with family
-and on and on...

We are thankful for you and send our love to you and your families.
12/1/14 Holidays... Holidaze

Thanksgiving has always meant the start of the holiday season for our family; this year as well although our personal circumstances are exceptional. We know of many close to us whose holidays have been turned upside down by tragedy, deployment, heartache, and any number of unforeseen situations, but this year we feel it far more deeply and daily. Our emotions have been up and down all week and we know we're not alone—feelings of comfort, anticipation and exhilaration alternating with sadness, loneliness and displacement.

Wonderful family time at Kim and Kevin's definitely met our need for togetherness (and time away from the rehab). We were there on Thanksgiving and again on Saturday for the Gator/FSU game (which brought other emotions to the surface). Friday was a pretty full therapy day for Dale, but Sunday was tough on both of us. Sometimes, a variety of factors just combine to leave a hollow place in our hearts and tears well up far too easily (and we've chosen not to hold them back). Dale and I are uprooted from our home and all that is familiar, even living apart from each other; saying goodbye to each other every night and sleeping alone definitely wears on us. It's been two months of that unforeseen practice and we don't know when that will end. So, we cry separately and together, revisit the reasons we are thankful for the care and rehab Dale is getting, and count the many blessings that we do have every day.

We KNOW we are where we belong, yet look forward to the day that we'll both be home. Thank God for victories, Dale's progress, our health, love and care of family, and friends who encourage.

It's hard to express how much your notes and cards mean to us both; they are read whenever our hope needs a boost, or we can use a reminder of the truths you share. Visits with family and friends are priceless treasures that we can look forward to and look back upon. Thank you.

We pray God's rich blessings on you and your families during this holiday time; every family is touched with the realities life brings; we pray joy and peace for each of you in the midst of life's trials.

> **NOTE: Truly, count your blessings, small or few as they may be at any given time. Voicing those out loud can change the atmosphere for all involved. There are always blessings; challenge yourself to look for them or start a thankfulness journal together, listing three each day. I encourage you to take that time; do it often, even repeatedly during the day. Your spirits will be lifted.**

12/6/14 Looking Forward...

We've had a good week and have marked progress in many ways, always needing specifics to review when progress seems slow. We have met with counselors, reviewed and reset Dale's therapy schedule, worked out respite days for Donna, and even had a wonderful day at the park with our grandsons. Dale has successfully discontinued one sleep medication, increased his physical workouts, mastered new sounds in speech, had several encouraging visitors this week and had his first outing with a friend and a staff member to watch football at TGIFriday's - without me! For each of these steps, we are most thankful, and we continue to rely on God's direction, grace for each moment, and peace in our hearts and minds.

Early this week, Dale's speech therapist discussed with us the possibility of intensive speech therapy as a next step. We've known that at some point Dale would need to move on, and yet with the stroke having directly affected the Broca's area (language center), he's experienced severe aphasia and apraxia. Recovery is a process that is multifaceted and often grueling, yet his/our focus is on complete recovery of speech and language understanding and usage as well as complete recovery from the stroke damage. This has been the goal from the beginning and has not changed.

> *Truly, count your blessings, small or few as they may be at any given time. Voicing those out loud can change the atmosphere for all involved.*

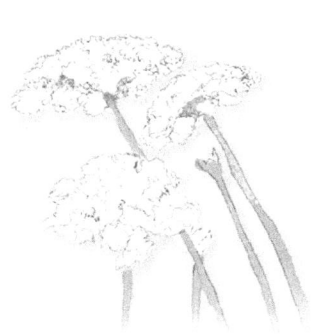

We were blessed to have already (before the stroke) studied research together on the neuroplasticity of the brain and the growing scientific awareness of the brain's awesome design and amazing ability to reroute neural pathways; our brains are constantly changing.

Here are some of the facts before us; we ask for your feedback, info, resources, help, and prayer:

-intensive speech therapy programs are available, but relatively few options; they are expensive and last 4-8 weeks; most often not covered by insurance; require much time and research on my part; most are far from our home.

-there are many options for online therapy and apps for all aspects of speech and brain recovery; reviewing and discerning those that will best help Dale is a daunting task in light of Dale's ability to utilize any of these options.

-we can't gauge how Dale's motivation will be for continued improvement if it is left up to his initiative; if I need to oversee and instruct all or most of this as he returns home, it will require much help, actually a team of individuals to assist in Dale's recovery and to assist and uphold us during a prolonged time of intense therapy. At this point, we do not know what this would look like.

-timing and finances are unknowns at this point. We are trusting that as one door closes, we'll know the next steps to take and are looking into options, rather blindly at this point.

As I've mentioned many times, God is our Refuge and God is our Strength, a very present help in trouble. He is in charge of our lives and His love and faithfulness to us are never ending and ever present. On that Truth we rest; it is our joy and peace to be in His loving care. We also know He has amazed us with orchestrating connections and situations that are so far beyond our thoughts and knowledge, we actually look forward to seeing how He provides the next step after NeuroRehab. In the meantime, we are fully engaging in what He has for us here and interacting with those He has placed in our lives. Dale is now assisting three individuals with workout/exercise programs and has two others waiting for health/nutrition discussions with him (with my help); we are involved with giving into the facility through upcoming teaching opportunities and regular feedback; I am helping several hours a week as a volunteer, and we are family to the patients and staff here as they allow us, especially during this Christmas season when emotions tend to be fragile.

In the midst of it all, we are grateful for time with Kim, Kevin, Richard, and Kate, and so very thankful for our longstanding good relationships and cherishing time together. God is good.

12/13/14 Update

It's hard for me to believe that it's been a week since I've updated. All is well and Dale continues to show much improvement. We just finished our fifth week at NSF, so this week has been filled with evaluations, meetings and adjustments. I've had long, busy days and am thankful to sleep well at night and for the opportunity to exercise regularly. Monday, December 8th, was my first full respite day, leaving Dale and the rehab at 6:00 p.m. on Sunday and returning Tuesday morning. I've been able to implement this now that his schedules are established, and we both trust the staff to handle anything that arises. Dale has been sleeping well since we arrived here, a real blessing for all and a boon to his recovery in every way.

Here are a few of the highlights this week:
- new NSF administration implemented beneficial changes
- Dale's evaluations are all positive and continue to show progress; he is about finished with PT
- speech therapy will be increasing to twice daily
- our concerns and requests are heard and discussed; appropriate changes are in process
- Dale is replying to questions in short, complete sentences—a big step—and all staff is implementing that practice
- dermatology appt. was comfortable; nurse practitioner was thorough, caring, and conscientious - a good experience
- we had visits from hometown friends, Christy and our friend who is working with Dale on brain health evaluation and exercises; we are blessed by this and grateful she's studied brain health for the last two years
- Dale went to Thursday night football again with the "guys"
- he is singing a lot and we have been singing together when I play the keyboard (we keep it in his room)
- I was able to surprise him today with the TSO concert in downtown Tampa; they are favorites of ours- a great concert!

-we were blessed with a HUGE financial gift that will pay forward to cover the cost of our insurance deductible and out of pocket maximum for 2015!!!

NOTE: It's important to note here that I prepared for the concert as well as I knew how. Dale wore a lanyard with his name on it telling of communication issues, and with my picture and phone number on the other side. And knowing the concert's volume would alone be highly stimulating, ear plugs were the plan. However, I left them in the car! So, I had to go to the First Aid station clear on the opposite side of the arena, leaving Dale in his seat ALONE. *That was not part of the plan.* **However, circumstances are likely (if you choose to be in any arena situation) that you might need food or drink, so it is worth considering the best plan—to leave him alone OR to face the crowds and long line. Just important to consider as you plan. By the way, I explained the situation and the timeframe carefully to Dale and that there was much for him to engage in while I was away. Thankfully Dale did fine, but I was on high alert!**

At times, emotions still run very high, and Dale's frustration quickly surfaces with not being able to communicate as he'd like. Of course, progress is slower than he wants and he's also hearing himself with better recognition. That brings self-correction (good) but also higher frustration when he can't make the sounds he wants. This is hard for both of us and can escalate quickly; we are meeting with the doctor this week to learn more about the moods caused by traumatic brain injury (TBI) and options for help. Much more to learn...

I praise God for His faithfulness in guiding us day by day, for our good sleep and good energy levels, for sunshine and beautiful weather, for continued progress and bountiful blessings. These are the things that keep us moving forward, even though sometimes we feel like we're barely trudging along. Your prayers buoy us, your caring means more than we can express and often brings out grateful tears. I'll update when time permits; only God knows my schedule.

12/20/2014 Happy Birthday to Me!

Dale and I planned a day out for my birthday but when I arrived this morning, he wasn't ready; in fact, it wasn't on his mind. He had been working hard of his own initiative to write out the alphabet and numbers from one to ten! Wow! This is a big first! When asked this past week, he had even told the doctor that he couldn't write. I'm impressed with his initiative, finding all the materials, persevering through the struggle, clarity of letters, using lined paper... complex thinking with great success. Many more neural pathways reconnected today! Later, when we were in Office Depot, he asked to find and purchase larger elementary lined paper and fine point Sharpies, so we did! Glad he plans to keep working on this.

Had a great day out—shopping, movie (Hunger Games Mockingjay), haircut, dinner, and Christmas light show synced to TSO music. It was a full day that showed Dale's increased endurance with no confusion or frustration. Great birthday gift to me.

Although everything was what we normally would have done on a day like today, when I asked if doing normal things outside of rehab all day gave him opportunity to feel normal, he said "no". Although non-speaking times were many, he was still hampered by speech in conversing with the barber and the waitress and sometimes in getting thoughts across to me. And, of course, we had to return to rehab is never his choice; however, he graciously didn't prolong discussion of it. We are grateful for this outing in beautiful weather doing things we enjoy together and thankful he is well and capable to do so.

Tomorrow, we spend the day at Kim's for her family Christmas and look forward to time all together. God is good and we are blessed.

12/27/2014 Home for the Holidays

Well, it's been said many a time that there's no place like home for the holidays and, wow, does that ring true for us this year! We had been able to anticipate this visit for over a month, bringing hope and a foreseeable goal. We started Sunday afternoon at Kim and Kevin's with Kate and Richard—relaxing, great food, and watching a few movies. Then on Christmas Eve, we headed to Englewood. Dale passed every milestone for this trip with flying colors. He endured the 1½ hours in the car peaceably, visited our condo for a couple of hours (a first in over three months), kept a reasonable, balanced schedule, slept the whole night, and made it back to rehab, although it was emotional. This ensures we can have more overnights.

We were blessed by our family gathering at David's Christmas Eve. Our family from Sarasota were with us, Steph cooked David's venison to perfection, everyone brought great food, all three boys played Christmas carols and other favorites on their new piano, and cousin Michelle treated us all to an impromptu concert, heart-warming and inspirational to the boys. Christy, Dale, and I stayed overnight at David's and it was precious to all be under one roof.

These are a few of our favorite things:
- Caleb and Gramma watching sunrise on the front porch
- the boys crawling in bed with Papa to wake him
- hot chocolate station up and running early
- breakfast of quiche Christy and the boys had made and our cranberry cheese bread
- Aunt Christy in her Gator Santa hat and PJs playing Santa
- smiles all around and lots of laughs, too…priceless!

It's the simple things that are such a blessing:
- a touch on the shoulder
- morning hugs

-sitting in the same room together
-familiar sights, sounds, and aromas
-memories recalled
-Christmas carols heard from several rooms; Papa joining in.

As with most gatherings, challenges occurred and were overcome. David and Stephanie's Christmas present of new countertops left them without a kitchen sink for those few days. Paper goods and bottled water came to the rescue along with dishwashing in the tub or outside (a new experience); Donna was battling a bug of some sort so Patti and Bill came to rescue Dale from rehab and deliver him to the family (they were rewarded with Dale's air guitar to TSO on the drive down); Donna recovered to lead carols on Christmas morning with Christy's able assistance and to enjoy family dinner before heading back to Tampa.

These inconveniences are the basis for growth and cooperation, patience, and kindness toward others, and will be the underpinnings of new memories, with only the sweet fragrance remaining. It is when we feel inconvenienced or neglected or in any way sorry for ourselves that we would be wise to look outward, to give to others, to glimpse the bigger picture and put our relatively minor trials in perspective. We live free; we are loved; we are fed and clothed and sheltered; we have so much for which to be thankful. Consider those who live under tyranny, without loved ones or knowledge of God's love, without food, clothing, or shelter; pray for their needs to be met and ask how we can be involved, and for them to know that God is as close as their breath, hears their every sigh, holds them close to His heart, and loves them beyond measure.

We are blessed and count it a great joy to have had this Christmas time. Our prayer for you, dear friends, is that our Father God gives you wisdom, hope, revelation and enlightenment, joy, and encouragement in the name of Jesus so that you may know Him better and the plans He has for you. May you look forward to 2015 as a precious gift of time and cherish the relationships you have, remembering the very fragility of life. We love you.

12/29/2014 Realigning

I'm thankful many things have been chronicled in Caring Bridge for future pondering. As I'm encouraged by truth and the real-life stories of others, I am reminded of my part which is to help, come alongside of, build up, and encourage Dale *in his faith*. In this practice, I have fallen short. There are reasons, some seem like excuses, but the reality is that I need to realign my focus.

"I will be your God through all your lifetime. I made you and will care for you. I will carry you along and be your Savior." Isaiah 46:4

It's one thing to know this for myself and be encouraged, but when Dale needs help even to read or concentrate, it is my privilege to be there to remind and encourage him in Truth. Help me, Lord.

1/6/2015 Happy New Year

Wow, since Christmas, we have been on the go! As usual, the lack of routine set off by the holidays has kept us wondering what day it is. We've kept a full schedule and Dale's endurance and energy level has been strong. Hallelujah!

Here are some highlights:
- we enjoyed sharing gifts with our rehab friends and staff
- Dale is copying letters/numbers with accuracy and clarity
- his reading has improved
- a friend came up from Naples to visit and watch football
- Dale is now able to button shirts readily, after only two tries
- he has successfully shaved with his electric clippers

-we spent all New Year's Day at Kim and Kevin's, staying late to enjoy the family fun as Oregon trounced FSU

-Dale is assisting with household tasks as a part of OT, things he has normally done around the house

-he made a grocery list for his breakfast project and completed the shopping with his occupational therapist

-Christy and best friend came for the weekend; went to Gator Dockside for the Gator game, then movies and a long walk at Wiregrass Shops followed by dinner at a local Vietnamese restaurant; we all stayed overnight at nearby hotel...

-then David's family joined us for a full day at Busch Gardens, celebrating the birthdays of two grandsons on the last day of vacation

We're so grateful to be able to have overnights! Even though there have only been two so far, it's a great encouragement to see progress that moves us homeward. When time drags by slowly at the rehab, or communication is frustrating, or when we still have to say goodbye for the evening, these are the things that bring hope and remind us of progress.

Thank you for your consistent encouragement and the holiday emails, cards and calls; we are blessed to have your help in lifting our spirits. In the of midst our present situation, we are mindful of the life trials of others who also need healing and encouragement and lift them in prayer. We are not alone; we all need each other.

Chapter Four

PREPARING FOR HOME

1/12/15 Good News!

Expected discharge date from rehab January 31. In just under three weeks we'll be home! Dale is relieved and filled with anticipation. Donna is making lists and checking them twice, listening for good counsel, watching plans begin to unfold, and moving forward step by step. Big changes are in the making and we need your prayers, resources, and support.

This week, Dale was evaluated by the director of a cutting-edge online speech therapy clinic and will be taking online speech sessions weekly during January, adding a second session after we get home. We are thrilled with this man's expertise, years of experience, innovation, and dedication. Dale has been excited about this possibility since we first spoke by phone in mid-December. It certainly has given us direction as we plan toward coming home.

Other progress for Dale this week included:
- cooking breakfast - safely chopping vegetables and using stove, toaster, and coffeemaker
- maintaining focus in a crowd
- strengthening fingers on guitars (uncertain of chords yet)
- shaved with clippers successfully for second time
- improved dexterity with jacket zippers
- began silently reading hard copy along with audiobook

In addition, we spent the first overnight in our condo (in over three months) and all went well with sleeping, schedules, and expectations. We do realize that Dale will not be left alone, nor will he venture forth from the house alone. We'll need a support team as we move home. Please pray for continued direction and peace, healing, and renewal of Dale's brain functions and connections. We are grateful that he has been restored in so many areas so quickly and thank God for wisdom and healing.

> *Simplify decisions.*
> *Take things slowly;*
> *pause when needed;*
> *take deep breaths*
> *and encourage*
> *others to as well.*

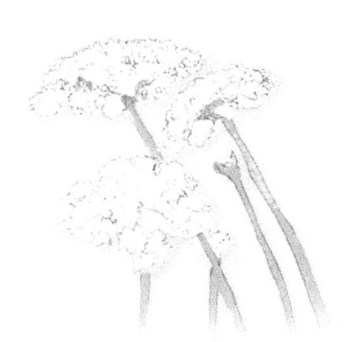

1/20/15 Update

We had a great weekend at home! It was filled with family, friends, and activities. Dale did great with everything and had his first online speech class with me and a good friend learning as coaches. This week, he will work on exercises for relearning keyboarding and for separating his vocalization from his jaw movement. It is extremely interesting! We are very blessed to be a part of this online learning opportunity; however, it is not a normal part of our insurance coverage so please pray for favor as we bring it to the insurance case manager.

Dale passed his swim test as expected and is just as comfortable as he always was in the pool. He is now working on dexterity with using a knife at his meals and operating scissors.

Our conversations about returning home are that we are not afraid, but cautious. It is going to be very different with me being the only one speaking to him about what to do—always a challenge for this wife, even in normal circumstances! We have had wise counsel as to how to word things in a positive way without issuing a command; now please pray that will become my practice quickly.

We are continually grateful for Kim and Kevin and the relationship that we have. Their care for me has been loving and continual. Once again this morning, my heart is grateful for them both as Kim sent a care package to the rehab clients and Kevin directed me to the best place to get my tire fixed. (I found that I had the second nail in the same tire since I've been in Tampa!) As I write this entry, I am waiting for that tire to be patched before getting on the highway for my day with Dale. This weekend, we look forward to more time with family and friends, staying at Kim and Kevin's, and going to a movie.

It was pointed out to us that this time away from rehab is good for everyone involved – us to be away and involved in normal socializing, and for the staff and patients at the rehab to be weaned from our daily presence before we 'disappear' altogether.

Much is still to be done before we return home. We are taking one step at a time and grateful for God's direction at every turn.

1/27/2015 Reality Check

With four days left before Dale is discharged and we head home, I am faced with the reality of changes to which we will be adjusting after nearly four months of 24/7 professional care. Thoughts of being basically on my own with the responsibility of Dale's post-stroke needs are daunting, but as tears and fears threaten to overwhelm me, I am also gently reminded by the Spirit of God of His care, His truth, and my need for yielding to His greatness. That the Creator, the Master of the entire universe, knows me by name, loves me, and has promised to never leave me or forsake me brings peace to my mind and gives me a place to rest. I do not have to strive, to control, but to lean in and listen for direction moment by moment, thankful for loving family and wise counsel, both near and far.

"For my thoughts are not your thoughts, neither are your ways my ways," declares the LORD. As the heavens are higher than the earth, so are my ways higher than your ways and my thoughts than your thoughts." Isaiah 55:8-9

"Therefore, do not worry about tomorrow, for tomorrow will worry about itself. Each day has enough trouble of its own." Matthew 6:33

"Do not be anxious about anything, but in everything, by prayer and petition, with thanksgiving, present your requests to God. And the peace of God, which transcends all understanding, will guard your hearts and your minds in Christ Jesus." Philippians 4:6-7

As of Sunday, we began our goodbyes; Dale first saying goodbye to his sister and brother-in-law. Then we both said goodbyes to our weekend nurse. Today, we made an Appreciation Lunch for those with whom we've lived for the past three months and gave them our contact information with great hopes that we will be able to stay in touch. More of this to come Thursday, Friday, and Saturday.

Great changes for both of us as this NeuroRehab staff have ministered loving care and imparted great knowledge to each of us on a daily basis. They have taught and spoken wisdom to Dale. As we go home, much of that teaching and encouragement will come from me; I can only trust God will provide others to come alongside me to teach and support, that Dale will not only have my voice speaking to him daily. We have already had several offers to help in various ways and for that we are both so grateful; we really do see the beginnings of Team Dale coming together.

Yet, as my voice becomes the predominant one Dale hears on a daily basis, I pray for grace that it brings peace, hope and love as well as truth, wisdom and direction. Please pray that along with us and that we will move slowly, stay flexible in schedule and routine as needed, work hard, rest well, appreciate all we have, and enjoy each day.

1/28/2015 A Call for Help

> **NOTE: Although this entry is only a list of needs, I've included it here in original form so all the needs are detailed for any reader to consider in light of their personal situation.**

Many of you have offered help, and now we are ready for your help. Below is the list of present needs; they will change as we progress. If you are available to help, please contact us as soon as possible (email is best) with how and when you might be able to help, and we'll be in touch. THANK YOU IN ADVANCE.

FOOD - Meals have been taken care of for the first week. As we focus on restoration and brain health, our diet is very specific. Cooks/grocery shoppers should be familiar with Zone or Paleo food planning; gift cards are helpful from Publix, Reid's Nutrition, Richard's, Trader Joe's, and Whole Foods.

THERAPY COACHES - Dale needs at least three hours of language therapy six days a week, brain exercises daily, gym workouts three times a week, pool sessions, and walking three to four times weekly. We have training sessions available for speech and brain exercises; right now, his gym workouts need transportation and one-on-one supervision at the YMCA.

GUITAR - Dale has been a very good rhythm guitar player for decades and is interested in reconnecting those skills. Two recent sessions with a guitar-playing friend have shown us that his hand positions are correct and that he can visually follow a few simple chords when someone else is playing with him. However, he needs more playing time to help restore the cognitive brain connections to "hear" the chords and to recognize the visual music language (some of this involves the same process as he is working on with speech). Please let us know if you play guitar and have some time to help.

TRANSPORTATION/ACTIVITIES - Dale cannot drive, so will need transportation to the Y for workouts and social activities apart from Donna. We are also requesting transportation to high school sports events, Rays' games, etc.

COMPANION - Donna has been advised to take a respite day each week, so Dale will occasionally just need a companion when family members aren't available to spend all or part of that day with him.

MISCELLANEOUS - If your talent is administration/organization, we need someone to help manage Dale's therapy schedule. We are also looking for someone to do some occasional housecleaning.

Chapter Five

HOME SWEET HOME

2/7/2015 First Week Home!

Well, this first week has been FULL—full of unpacking, full of emotion, full of busyness and adjustments. It is SO good to be home, to settle into familiar surroundings, sleep in our own bed, set our own schedule, and make even little decisions.

Saturday, January 31st, I arrived at the rehab after an early morning goodbye to Kim and Kevin. Dale was packed and ready to head home! We arrived back in Englewood in time for grandson Matthew's basketball game... and things haven't slowed down much since then! David's family came over after lunch and Christy surprised us with a visit, too; Patti and Bill, Joshua, and a coaching friend came over to train as speech coaches, Patti cooked some meals while Bill and Christy went bridge-walking with Dale. Dinner was on the porch at sunset, a wonderful end to our first day back.

It is a blessing that the time at NeuroRehab set Dale's biological clock, which in turn helped him have enough rest to encourage healing. His energy is great and has been tested throughout January as we embarked on various outings, including a Busch Gardens day.

Dale's first question/concern was, "What if it happens again?" So, our fire medic friend who played football with David and was coached by Dale spent time with us reviewing Dale's medical info sheet and sharing info on local EMS procedures and hospitals.

Gaining that knowledge answered all of Dale's questions about emergency health care at home and brought peace to us all.

Then, thanks to a 6:30 p.m. game time, we got to enjoy the Super Bowl in the comfort of our own living room and still basically keep to Dale's schedule.

Over the past three months, Dale's body has basically had a reset in most ways; our goal is to maintain what now has become his normal circadian rhythm, brain healthy nutrition, and exercise. We expect to have little variation during this first month home, resting in the familiar. Also, during this month, we will move into therapies as soon as we have the opportunity, in some cases dependent upon insurance, hoping to develop a schedule once things line up.

This week, Dale has worked out at the YMCA three times (with a workout partner), attended grandsons' wrestling practice and basketball games, met out of town friends for lunch, attended the monthly breakfast of the Lemon Bay HS retired teachers where we reconnected with many supportive friends, and went to an evening church gathering. On Thursday, a friend took Dale for about five hours to workout, lunch, walk, and watch football shows! It was a test of faith for both of us (and likely for our friend as well). Tonight, Saturday, we and the grandsons met friends in Old Englewood Village for the best car show Dale and I have ever been to. It was totally enjoyable. Mexican food and *The Phantom Menace* movie finished off a nice time together.

Communication has continued to be our primary challenge, but we have been able to work things through or know they are to be dealt with later on. There have been intense "discussions," moments of frustration, lots of unpacking and resettling, research for anything that will help Dale move toward complete restoration, and of course, engaging on the phone for hours with insurance.

Bringing our concerns to Father has brought peace and direction; waiting on answers helps us to move slowly and circumspectly. We have many others for whom we are praying and our needs pale in light of some of their situations. I am glad Father knows what is best, and Holy Spirit is faithful to lead us; we are the ones who need to continue to turn to Him. Know we are well, enjoying each day and accomplishing with diligence what is set before us. We are blessed with beautiful weather, sunshine, fresh air, good rest, good food, peace, hope, and the love of family and friends as we move forward in this new phase of our life's journey.

2/17/2015 Honestly...

It's 3:42 a.m. and I've been awake since 12:30 a.m., having gone to sleep at 10:00 p.m. Nothing in particular is on my mind. I've journaled; I've prayed; I've read; I've nearly fallen asleep. It's an alone time and I've been feeling alone...in the midst of much doing. Sometimes, tears are a release; I ward off self-pity but am left with **the realization that it's me and Dale**. After months of 24/7 care, it's the two of us... and it's a HUGE adjustment. I can only imagine how Dale feels—alone in his thoughts, not who he was, not who he wants to be. That puts my aloneness in perspective, and I immediately am moved to pray for him and to consider his needs. I love the word *consider*. In Latin, it means **to view attentively, to sit by**;[2] when we truly sit by someone and view them attentively, we learn much.

Lord, help me as I help Dale and *consider* what steps to take. Let me sit by You, Lord, and be attentive, learning more about Who You are. You are Provider, Counselor, Peace, Life, Truth, Love, Wisdom, and All in All. Time considering You is the best way to spend the

---

[2] (American Dictionary of the English Language n.d.)

time You've given me, day or night; thank You that You never sleep, and I can rest in that truth and in Your help always.

I lift up my eyes to the hills-- where does my help come from? My help comes from the LORD, the Maker of heaven and earth. He will not let your foot slip-- he who watches over you will not slumber.
Psalm 121:1-3

2/17/2015 Changes

If change means growth, we are growing! Daily changes in schedule and therapies, even choices and attitudes make our life a constant challenge. Change is good for the brain, we understand. There is no plateau, no norm; our constant **is** *change*. Fortunately, our center is in God alone, He Who never changes. What a comfort, refuge, place of peace. Thank You, Father.

Dale's communication improves daily although it's like we're both learning a new language. It is a blessing to see that he is now most often careful to think before he tries to speak, choosing most important words and forming them as best he can. There are more and more times that he spontaneously voices understandable phrases, like "all sorts of things," that are totally clear. The language is still there inside, and he is so pleased when it comes out. So, we have times of rejoicing and much laughter as we work to understand what he's wanting to communicate. Although frustration is minimal, it does try to surface, and he needs to be reminded to relax, to do something else, and that frustration is not what we choose.

My sense of being overwhelmed tends to come from the overseeing, from the many small responsibilities, and the activity/therapy monitoring. I truly cannot do this alone and am thankful for those who pray for us and encourage us.

We now have a volunteer coach who is coming a few times a week, to work on speech and keyboarding with Dale; we pray she is blessed by this time as we are. This week he has three online speech sessions with his teacher/therapist, a remarkable man who's been involved with helping those with aphasia since 1976. In addition, last week we went to Naples to meet with two wonderful ladies, an OT and wellness trainer respectively, who are now working to assess Dale's needs and design therapies to specifically help him with motor skills, neural reconnection, and brain/nervous system health. We are MOST grateful to trust them, and it is our pleasure to call them friends. Time in Naples gives us opportunity to visit Christy as well; she actually was able to come to last week's session and we were pleased to spend some time at her softball practice that afternoon.

Our wellness trainer introduced us to the Stephen Jepson movement website (see Appendix One); we bought his DVD and spoke with him by phone. His message of movement and play is for everyone. At his recommendation we read *"Sitting Kills, Moving Heals"* by Dr. Joan Vernikos, former Director of NASA's Life Sciences Division, whose research on astronauts brought new knowledge to movement and aging. We are pleased to recommend this short book for **everyone**.

Those who have never been associated with traumatic brain injury or any other life altering situation cannot fathom how important normal social contact can be. We have noted for years that families who have met challenges of this sort (that cause a person to be considered "out of the norm") are blessed with more compassion and consideration. I first saw it as a child when my brother had a grave speech impediment throughout much of his elementary school experience. Children were cruel and adults were at a loss as to how to respond so they most often ignored or looked away. Years later, Dale and I both observed this social anomaly while teaching high school, specifically recognizing maturity and kindness in students of all ages who lived with a challenged family member. In addition, with my grandparents and Dale's mom, we learned that no matter what the state of the body is, the spirit is whole and eternal and is always in a position of receiving - both positive or negative input. *How quick our society judges according to perceived beauty and apparent knowledge, without taking time to listen or look deeper.* Now, here we are, with Dale looking "normal" but the perception quickly changes as he expresses himself. I've stated many times that we are learning, not only stroke/brain/therapy knowledge, but learning volumes about humankind, our Creator and His design (our bodies) and His plan for relationship with one another (1 John).

We are thankful for new mercies every morning, beautiful weather, a friend who did some ironing for us, wonderful therapy sessions, music, good rest, times of play, attending a dual piano concert, our friend's improved health (and his haircut for Dale!), Englewood Farmer's Market, gift cards, and Caring Bridge. We pray for those who are battling trauma and for their caregivers and families.

2/20/2015 Settling In…?

Often asked if I/we are settling in to being home, a new routine or schedule, I do weigh my response, wanting to be honest and not simply rhetorical. We ARE settling in and love being at home, but there is no schedule per se and, actually, our "new" life is just life… with new factors. Although they are rather major factors (Donna's retirement, Dale's recovery from stroke), we've had enough life experience to know that changing factors are simply LIFE, the life process.

Our best "settling in" is nesting and resting in God's plan for our life, abiding in Him minute by minute (our human challenge) and trusting His direction for our every need. When we can settle in with God, the external factors are simply the weather of each day, stormy or calm, sunny or grey; He remains the same, our Rock, our Father Who takes our hand when we can't see the way or carries us when we are exhausted or hurt or the road is too hard.

Are we settled in? Yes, secure in our Father's love, His timing, His wisdom that stretches far beyond what we can even imagine. Unrest simply causes us to seek Him more, on our knees before Him. Isn't that really where we belong?

2/23/2015 Sail On, Silver Girl

Yesterday morning, I was contemplating the possibility of writing a book—not for now, but so many have suggested that I should. However, for me, that could become a vain undertaking, so I was just taking this to my Father. Immediately, I felt that He would preserve me in the writing, and that our story could help others who are troubled in similar circumstance. The song *"Bridge Over Troubled Waters"* came to mind. We have always loved that song since Simon and Garfunkel recorded it. In the 70s I think it was singer Sammy Hall who first spoke of Jesus as that Bridge. As I sang it aloud and then looked up lyrics, realizing I had left out a verse, it became evident to me that this recollection was an encouragement from God of His presence in hard times. I was moved to tears by the reference to "sail on, silver girl." It can't get much more personal to me with my long silver hair at this stage of my life!

I further was reminded of a time in Naples when our pastor spoke over me regarding sailing, so I looked it up in my journal. "2006 - I'm in a small boat, rowing faithfully and consistently, yet the doing, the propulsion is mine. God is putting a sail on my boat, and He will fill the sail. I am to put down the oars and let the wind carry the boat." **God provides the wind**. My journaling that day was reflective of an act of the will, a line drawn in the sand—put off/cast off criticism and any tendency to manipulate circumstances or people. And... NOT to step into the place of the Holy Spirit to get in the way of what He is doing. So, I have put aside my "good" ideas of needed help, specific help from others. In doing so, I recognized a subtle manipulation, a reaction to fear, but when recognized, so obviously a device of the enemy to divert my efforts to "doing" instead of waiting and listening. So, I wait... and listen. "Sail on, silver girl," put down the oars, and float as He fills the sails.

Interesting that both of my 2014 journals, one I bought and one that Carol gifted me, are entitled "Trust in the Lord". Since the 70s, I've acknowledged Proverbs 3:5-6 as one of my life scriptures *"Trust in the Lord with ALL your heart and lean not unto your own understanding. In ALL your ways acknowledge Him and He WILL direct your paths."* Amen! Thank you, Daddy, for keeping me on track. (And, even as I write in this journal, I'm noting that another of my life Scriptures is printed as encouragement on this page: *"Seek first the Kingdom of God and His Righteousness, and all these things will be added unto you." Matthew 6:33*)

3/3/2015 A Month At Home

This past Saturday, February 28th, marked four weeks since we've been home. A pattern is developing for our weeks, and we've had time to reflect—on ourselves, on our perspectives, on God's workings in our lives, and on others. As I sit on the porch this morning overlooking the river and taking in the beauty of God's handiwork, I am conscious of feeling protected, away from the maelstrom, the rat race of the world. Since the stroke, our focus has been to hear and do what will bring Dale to complete recovery. That is so unlike what our lives had been up until October 3rd, 2014; we were always immersed in the goings-on of life, often on the frontlines leading and teaching others. Now, to be introspective, even self-protective, and to know that this time was set aside for that purpose, causes me to wonder: how long, what will be learned, what is our purpose, how to touch others. We've learned not to try to make things happen but to trust God both in times of activity and inactivity, yet to see the needs of others, to hear of happenings worldwide, makes me question what I should be <u>doing</u>. Dale is not questioning these things at this point; I'm not even sure they cross his mind. He is deeply focused on gaining normalcy in every aspect of his life. So, I take these musings to God and rest in His timing and plan for us; each of us have a personal walk and I am not to ever compare mine to others, but to be content. I am.

In so many ways, Dale has made great gains and, to watch him from a distance, most would not even know he had a stroke. That evidence shows in his speech, following instructions, sequencing, and directionality. We notice new brain reconnections nearly every day and are thankful for that; his whole being works very hard to accomplish what used to be automatic. I can't even imagine the energy output it takes for him to accomplish what is set before him.

This week, we venture out to have an overnight at Christy's, our first overnight away from home; we are praying for good rest for us both. Tampa Bay Rays' Spring Training games start tomorrow. We have tickets for all home games this month; the stadium is only a five-minute drive from our house. We are looking forward to baseball, getting to know the "new" team, and being outdoors in this beautiful weather. Planning to "work" on scorecards at each game. Also, we've been asked to attend an OT class at FGCU to have a discussion with OT students on therapy from a family and client perspective; we are thrilled to be able to help and LOVE working with students. March has a full calendar!

Dale's progress of the last ten days:
    -speaking three to four word sentences multiple times a day
    -many correct words now and new ones daily; he is so pleased to hear himself when say a word correctly

-after three weeks of waiting, insurance approved OT right here in town. The therapist is wonderful and highly recommended. Bonus is that there is a shuttle for Dale right to our front door! That gift just redeemed a couple of hours for me twice a week and gives him a measure of independence/time without me.

-Dale is regularly making breakfast for us

-moving forward in brain exercises with success

-advancing in speech therapy in spurts, working on consonants and blends. His teacher is pleased and so are we.

-he definitely thinks hard before speaking - we could all benefit from applying that wisdom!

-he definitely is grateful to exercise his opinions and choices, something he was limited in until we got home. We try to go with those as often as possible.

-self-generated writing and spelling a word for the first time

-got first three letters written before getting stuck; I was able to guess the word and consequently the topic

-continues to engage socially, with known acquaintants and new ones alike; relies on my help but not fearful.

-take short walks around our condo neighborhood by himself

-together we're reading *"Return to Ithaca,"* a stroke survivor's account of her recovery after a severe stroke, very in-depth perspective.

-after therapy in Naples, spent the evening with Christy and best friend - so heartwarming to enjoy an evening with them

-dinner and watching American Idol had been a weekly tradition for us for years while living in Naples, a time to catch up together. Felt normal, at least to me.

Challenges:

-Dale is remembering things that happened in the first month after the stroke. We can only discuss them in part as he really can't ask or tell details yet. I usually tell him what I know in order to bring clarity and truth into the picture, then we have to put it aside until his communication is better.

-he is often impatient when I don't understand things we've talked about before; usually there is no context for me to reference at these times. I remind him of that and ask him to be patient with me in this, too.

-left and right still are not clear; it's clearly more frustrating to me than to him at this point

-not a lot of rational thinking on his part, but we do see it surface, sometimes in surprising circumstances

-limited perception of others in the moment; however, when he's relaxed, he does express concerns he has about others

-mindful that he can't drive and yet frustrated as he sees lousy drivers on the road all the time. Got a letter from DMV about it that brought it all to the surface again

Thank you for your continued care and prayer and for staying in touch. You make this long journey so much more bearable.

3/14/15 Normalcy...

Normalcy: a term often used indiscriminately, without thought, and we tend to readily agree with it... without thought as well.

This week, I've been aware of a few things that are "imposed" upon us by the expectations (usually ignorant) of others; there is a constant battle of the mind. We are bombarded daily by multitudes of beliefs (or "unbeliefs") that are spoken to us or over us with regularity, and yet have no foundation in actual truth or knowledge.

To bring this philosophizing down to our personal situation with Dale's recovery, we have to take every thought and word, no matter how well-meaning or how "expert" the speaker, and examine it according to God's Word, the Truth.

There is much "out there" that wants to limit recovery from stroke—misconceptions, traditional thinking, laziness, "expertise" and the desire to be "right," money, time, impatience... and the list continues. Insurance companies are a huge factor, and the high cost of adequate, specifically appropriate care looms like a giant. *Yet we are not satisfied with the commonplace but are seeking what will be Dale-specific.* We seek what is true and beneficial and reject the rest.

"We demolish arguments and every pretension that sets itself up against the knowledge of God, and we take captive every thought to make it obedient to Christ." 2 Corinthians 10:5

> ...we are not satisfied with the commonplace but are seeking what will be Dale-specific.

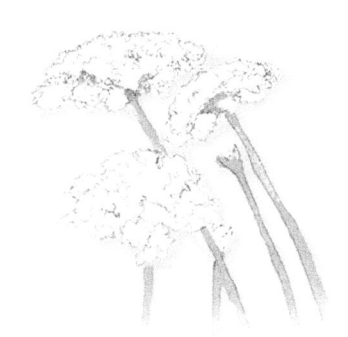

Our trust has to be in God's direction, His opening of doors, His provision for these needs, many of which we don't even know yet, but He does, and in that we can rest. I am so grateful that my Father addressed these concerns before I even knew them. *"So do not worry, saying, 'What shall we eat?' or 'What shall we drink?' or 'What shall we wear?' ...your heavenly Father knows that you need them. But seek first his kingdom and his righteousness, and all these things will be given to you as well. Therefore, do not worry about tomorrow, for tomorrow will worry about itself. Each day has enough trouble of its own."* Matthew 6:31-34

Blessings this week for which we are thankful:
- a new helper who contacted us "out of the blue"
- wise therapists who discuss needs and details, ask for feedback, to make adjustments specifically designed for Dale
- friends who help just because they know they have something helpful to offer
- good rest and good, healthy food
- opportunities to give to others
- spring training baseball for recreation and time outside
- our family - time spent with them in person or on the phone
- God's direction - presenting new possibilities and opening doors for us and for those we meet
- beautiful weather
- those who encourage and/or pray for us

Prayer requests:
- that we discern what is good for Dale and us, not taking the easier route but the one that is best for Dale
- for grace, strength, and protection as we travel to Miami for a balance/vision workshop; that we would set a good pace for learning and rest during the full days of sessions
- for those students/teachers we will meet with at FGCU on Wednesday that we may impart family and client feedback to enhance their learning how to help others
- for wisdom regarding travel this week and next month

Chapter Six

SIX MONTHS AND COUNTING

4/1/15 Six Month Update

We've been home for two months now and Dale is six months into recovery. God is good and we have good reports to share.

Our workshop in Miami was wonderful and well-paced; we were able to attend all the sessions and get good rest at night. Hallelujah! The teacher is perceptive, dedicated, a good instructor, and truly cares about people. We got to tell our story and Dale was a guest "subject," willingly allowing himself to work with the teacher in demonstrations in front of the group of sixty attendees. I'm so proud of him for that willingness. We learned much, met new people, received encouragement and new resources, and are hoping to plan and host this Bal-A-Vis-X workshop in southwest Florida this fall.

Our discussion session at FGCU with first year OT students was a real pleasure for us. Both of our lives have been spent teaching and imparting to others; the self-care and focus on us since Dale's stroke has not been our norm, so it was a heartwarming to help others in their learning process as therapists. I shared details of our story for over an hour with a few intermittent questions, then Dale had a chance to talk. Although he simply said, "thank you" and "it's hard," the students then engaged him in Q&A which he handled comfortably, deferring to me whenever needed. There was no question we wouldn't answer; our goal was to share transparently as survivor and family so these future therapists could learn the personal side of the effects of stroke—traumatic, life-changing, scary, unknown, and un-prepared-for. It has become our belief that *anyone ministering to a stroke victim and their family should assume NOTHING but ask a series of questions and personal details so they can relate to their situation personally.* We were blessed to be a small part in their education.

March has been filled with other "normal" interactions as we attended many Tampa Bay Rays' spring training games, Caleb's baseball games, Christy's softball games, David's fishing tournaments, and had much social interaction with "snowbird" condo neighbors as well as family visits. Our weather has been outstanding, sunny with comfortable temperatures, so we've been able to keep the house open to the fresh breezes. This morning we'll attend a breakfast with retired teachers from Lemon Bay HS where Dale taught for twenty-four years. They are a treasury of friends.

Therapy-wise, Dale diligently works on over **fifteen** therapies at home, and still attends OT sessions twice a week and "brain" therapy once a week. He diligently works through these with me, by himself, or with a coach when she's available to help us. All four of his therapists remarked last week about his increased conversationality, confidence, and progress; we are thankful. It is hard work and Dale often says so when asked how he's doing. He takes needed breaks and rest, but, as many of you have testified to him, he is definitely a strong rehabber! In addition, he's begun getting up earlier so we can walk about forty minutes before the sun gets strong, and if we are watching TV in the evening, he gets up to use the Bosu ball during commercials. As of two weeks ago, he gets his day started by himself three mornings a week while I join neighbors at the clubhouse for line dance class, and we workout at the Y at least twice a week. This is total body therapy; no wonder he's moving forward so well!

However, that's not to say there aren't hard times. The trial of conversation can often be frustrating to both of us, and we share tears when the loss seems overwhelming, but in the big picture those times are relatively few. And... interaction with insurance has been a battle that I have to gear up for; please keep that in prayer.

We are grateful for:
- those who encourage us
- family and friends who will visit or invite us to join them
- wonderful, innovative therapies and therapists
- those who assist by coaching Dale
- being home and the healing place it is
- living on the river
- God's direction for each day and His comfort and peace
- farmers' markets
- David's fishing team's win in the first tourney of the season
- opportunity to watch Christy's co-ed softball team in Naples (we love/miss this)
- a good car and audiobooks for when we drive

4/12/2015 Perspective from My Porch

Taking in the early morning wonders from our back porch, I am at rest living on the Myakka River. I enjoy the rabbits, fresh air, boats, neighbors, staff, line dancing, bridge, pool, boat dock, clubhouse, and yard maintenance - all blessings that I don't take for granted.

So, I am filled, refreshed, **and** directed as I meditate on God and the added pleasure**, gift, and** inspiration of this porch environment in the early morning. Of course, like Peter the apostle who wanted to build three tabernacles and "camp" at the mount of transfiguration, in my humanness I too want to camp here or make this a permanent scheduled time... only leading to disappointment as things change and life happens. Lord, rescue me from my "self!"

For today, I'll note blessings in the midst of this trial, changes provoked by the stroke that brought some relief, rest, health and thankfulness for areas of concern that are resolved or better understood. Some are not pretty to discuss/consider and of which Dale was not cognizant, not addressing or struggling with unsuccessfully, but in reality, have been a cause for concern for us who love Dale:

- driving ability (he can no longer legally drive)
- alcohol – it's not allowed; he knows it adversely affects the brain. I'm grateful there's no resistance
- wholesome choices - are now my responsibility
- healthy, best brain food/supplements - he eats what I buy
- no testosterone supplements, which initially helped with depression after four joint replacements, but there were too many disadvantages
- system "reset" - much better digestion and sleep cycle
- improved self-worth, in many ways - not critical of himself
- memory issues are no longer considered a possibility; we know **for sure** memory is affected
- retirement adjustment is no longer a priority/concern
- complete health screening - we stay up to date on any issues and have great doctors

4/22/15 Each One's Experience is Unique

Talked at length last night with a new caregiver acquaintance whose husband also has aphasia. Everyone's story is SO different and I immediately began counting our blessings for the things we experienced that they did not. Thank you, Lord, for:

- us being together when Dale stroked, that he was not alone
- tPA administration being a viable option
- good doctors - everywhere we went
- my previous experience with patient and health advocacy
- early baseline MRI - a year before stroke

-Dale's excellent general health
-Dale's knowledge and understanding of the body and brain
-travel experience for both of us
-present social opportunities
-weather that is nice year-round so we can be outside
-NSF rehab and what we learned
-importance of scheduling and routine
-an SLP's example of working with Dale's frustrations
-staff's candid conversations with Dale re: my respite needs

So many need so much. That is why I need to tell our story - to help in any way. Every one's experiences can help.

5/3/15 A Real Vacation

Another month and we continue to move forward. The biggest improvement is in Dale's confidence to live life and interact with others. He's been encouraged by all his therapists from the onset of stroke, to do everything he thinks he should to establish his own "new normal." On occasion, he specifically tells me that very thing.

This month's update includes a REAL vacation. All went wonderfully well but it was a step-by-step process to make it happen. That's pretty much how our life has been, one step at a time; actually, a good and simple way of life.

> *-Flash back to October 3rd - I had just retired and we were heading up to Hilton Head to meet my sister Nancy and brother-in-law Ken, intending to take a week-long road trip ending in Gainesville for Dale's birthday and 45th Gator football reunion. On our first overnight at Amelia Island, Dale had the stroke and our vacation plans disintegrated. In the aftermath, I called to hopefully preserve our Hilton Head*

timeshare days and, after speaking to several levels of supervisors, was able to retain our days to use within a year.

During February, our first month home, I told Dale of these available vacation days and that it was opportune while Nancy and Ken still had some respite time. Well, Dale's first reaction was shock; in <u>his</u> mind Hilton Head = stroke! However, once he realized we would NOT go through Amelia Island, he agreed to pursue Hilton Head.

Dale had been cleared by his doctors back in January to travel by any means; however, he was initially wary to make any flight plans. By March, when a date had been reserved for Hilton Head, he decided to fly rather than drive. This would be a relatively short trip and I considered it a good first jaunt, with Nancy and Ken picking us up in Savannah and having their car available for the duration.

Packing was a well-thought-out process and I had to handle all of it so I would know where to find all of his belongings. Dale made clothing decisions; choices were kept to a minimum. He was glad to carry suitcases, although still a bit disoriented in finding handles and in the best way to load the trunk. He unpacked on his own, putting everything in drawers/closet; I only had to consolidate a bit to find things easily and, of course, still handled all meds and supplements.

All glory be to God, the One Who directs our path. *"Trust in the Lord with all your heart, and lean not on your own understanding; in all your ways acknowledge Him, and He shall direct your paths."*
Proverbs 3:5-6

Flight arrangements had been made for midday so we would have ample time to ready ourselves in the morning; we have learned that rushing is both unproductive and frustrating. A dear friend drove us and housed our car for the week. Airports were small, except the Atlanta transfer; Dale wore a bright-colored shirt so I could spot him easily. Next time, I will also wear something easily identifiable and identical for his sake and I will also take pics of each of us to put on each other's phones in case of separation (those things came to mind <u>as</u> we walked through Atlanta airport!).

We were blessed with great weather, a beautiful resort, lovely drives to Charleston and Savannah, awesome food at locals' favorite restaurants, and, of course, time with Nancy and Ken. Our history together is precious to all four of us and it was great for both Dale and me to have individual time away from each other for a couple of hours, not easy to do during this season of our lives.

As expected, this was a welcome break from therapy sessions and/or practices; although Dale chose to bring a few therapy tools, he hardly used them. Communicating, however, was a constant practice and he did a great job with Nancy and Ken, who were very patient and encouraging. We did have a lot of laughter as he shared how he could talk like a Wookie and sing like Bob Dylan!

Future trips are now in the making to Melbourne, Key West, Gainesville, even a few Rays' games at the Trop in St. Pete. A few weeks ago, Dale had come home from his OT shuttle and let me know he'd heard about local bus tours. We checked it out on the internet, asked lots of questions and found it to be a great option for us now, giving Dale no need to bemoan that "he'd have to all the <u>riding</u> while I have to do all the <u>driving</u>."

Thank you all who've been praying for us; we are well and dive back into therapy this week. Please write us about you and your families.

> **NOTE: To be perfectly honest, I experienced a few hours of second-guessing our decision to take this trip after a number of people were "surprised" we would travel, said I was "brave," etc. I'm sure at the time, those individuals**

had no idea they were imparting fear to me but it made me realize once again the power of our words and to think before I speak—a good reminder anytime. A few nights before we left, I woke up concerned with the wisdom of this venture. As I prayerfully asked God for direction, the next morning I received phone calls from dear friends and family encouraging me that they had been praying specifically for us and our trip.

Then, Saturday morning before our departure on Sunday, we awoke to find our AC not working; landlord called the tech who sadly told us the compressor was dead and couldn't even be ordered until Monday. *Perfect time for a vacation, right?* Plan B was activated, and while Dale was at our grandson's baseball game with David, I completed the packing and headed to spend the night with David's family by late afternoon. It was actually a blessing to have that all completed and the car packed early on. (The awesomeness of God was evident when, as we departed from Hilton Head the <u>following</u> Friday, we learned the compressor was finally being installed THAT VERY MORNING and house would be cool upon our arrival. The AC had not been functioning the entire time we were gone!)

5/20/2015 Seroquel Notes

Dale had been on Seroquel since November to help sleep at night so he could have good rest. Although it's an anti-psychotic, it was the only effective medication that helped him overcome anxiety during the hardest times after the stroke when his brain was still very inflamed/swollen. (I'm fully aware this is my description, not medically specific, but his brain was highly traumatized by the stroke, affecting vision, perception, understanding and critical thinking as well as speech and some motor functions.) His sleep and daily routine have been stable for several months.

As some of these areas noticeably recovered to varying degrees, we were looking for ways to bring more clarity to his speech therapy since Dale's greatest desire was to improve his speech. So, on May 4th, he dosed down from 50mg to 25mg. However, after ten days, we resumed full 50 mg dose after observing the following:
-Dale mentioned nightmares twice and also told his doctor
-he had been more "down"
-he had been frustrated more frequently

No other factors/changes had occurred in his life/routine except he was finished and discharged from OT so, consequently, had more freedom and choices of how to spend his time. Routine is comforting. Carol mentioned that the cumulative effects of Seroquel on two of her family members affected daytime behavior. Dale's sleep has not changed. Knowing that Seroquel is an antipsychotic and that he does deal with much anxiety post-stroke, we resumed the full dose. It took a few days for the cumulative effect to take hold. In the meantime, family noticed for a couple of days he was more distant, didn't initiate walks, didn't get dressed, didn't notice a piece missing from his hand gripper, and didn't smile much.

5/21/2015 Physical Setback as the "Real" Dale Shows Up

We had gone to help a church cleanup and, after about an hour, I think Dale overexerted himself carrying a heavy object a long way by himself (the "real" Dale kind of thinking kicked in). Dale told me something was wrong, and we left so we could talk in the car. He had a headache in his forehead, not sharp. We talked about his strength being good, but that his endurance was weakened. As Sam stated, "It's not a surprise that the 'real' Dale overdid something physical!" He was just living his life, I guess, and I try to let him. He is now recovering, laying low for a few days and we expect rhythm and stride to be restored. We are thankful for solid, normal sleep last night and a beautiful porch for pondering this morning. God's mercies are new every morning!

6/8/2015 Working Hard

Dale basically recovered and resumed therapy on the 27th, showing his normal interests. His motivation has improved but he also battles discouragement with communicating. That is hard for us both.

After a great first guitar lesson with our friend, Dale has worked regularly with guitar, building up his fingers. So glad to see it!

Today, however, he really struggled with speech exercises, reading sounds and words. He seemed to know it before starting. I had to work with him to help and encourage speech, but we made it. However, he gladly worked out, did balance balls, played guitar and walked. It's hard to write these things, but valuable to track changes.

7/1/15 Summer Weekends

Each day is a new opportunity to move forward, learn more and enjoy life. God is in charge of our lives and, although we'd like to see things move along faster, we do trust His wisdom and timing. Jesus rose from the grave and is seated at the right hand of the Father as King over all. We yield to His Lordship in our lives and are thankful for the comfort and guidance of his Spirit each day.

We had a family reunion right here in town mid-June and we're grateful to have had wonderful time with so many family members, up to forty of us, for three days. We are blessed that they traveled to us this year so we could continue our annual summer gatherings.

July will have us traveling every weekend and we'd love to see you, so let us know if we can get together while we're in your area. July 4-5 Siesta Key; July 10-12 Melbourne (dinner gathering with friends and music on July 11; let us know if you can join us in Palm Bay); July 18-19 Tampa/Brandon; July 24-26 Gainesville (FL) and then travel to north GA mountains July 27-29. Still at home weekdays and usually in Naples one day a week for therapy and to visit Christy.

We rely on your support during the tough times... and there are tough times, emotional and frustrating. I can't even imagine being in Dale's shoes and not being able to communicate what you want to say, especially when he is still so knowledgeable and spent his life teaching and helping others.

7/20/2015 Keep On Learning...

Well, we've had three weekends out of town that were both wonderful and enlightening.

First, a weekend at Siesta Key over the 4th of July, an excursion filled with walking on the shore and resistance walking in the water plus just sitting on the beach (under an umbrella, of course), but after four hours in the sun/heat, we were sapped. Dale went straight to the shower and crashed on the bed watching Wimbledon; I ordered out for brunch, walked to pick it up, then read an entire book. We love Siesta Key, enjoyed fireworks on the beach with Patti and Bill (who both biked over from home) and a couple of new friends. Very nice evening and no traffic to fight; we walked from our hotel!

Realizing that we were preparing for a month of weekends away, we kept basics in our suitcase and a cooler for the car, cutting back on prep time for the next trip—a big plus since most of that responsibility is now mine (another big adjustment that is now part of our new normal). Our visit to Melbourne began on July 10th, our

44th anniversary; we enjoyed a relaxed drive over with a great Clive Cussler audiobook and a lunch stop in Okeechobee for old times sake at Gladys' restaurant on the town square. We had been there many times with Dale's family on fishing weekends at their 'Gator Den' before we had kids. Home-cooked classics of Cobb salad and a meatloaf sandwich took us back in time...

We have such great friends! Our stay in Melbourne with Dale's high school friend was warm and welcoming with personal first-class accommodations at their home, then a great seafood meal as we overlooked the Indian River, a visit to the beach where he and Dale used to surf fish, a personal tour of his business, and then, his favorite frozen yogurt shop! The guys went fishing in the morning behind the house on the Indian River and later ran errands, driving around more familiar areas of town, a blessing for us both - Dale didn't have to only hear MY voice and I had cherished alone time.

Dinner with more friends Saturday was warm and memorable; ten of us around a square table with great food, LOTS OF STORIES, and great music by more of Dale's high school friends. These guys played together in a garage band when Dale was in high school and lived across the street! Beatles songs, original compositions, *Heart of Gold,* and everyone joining in to sing *You've Got a Friend...* priceless. We were even treated to an elementary school camp song by two friends from different towns. Go figure! Two guys represented both Dale's high school and Gator football teams; the stories flowed, and Dale was right in the midst of it all. He hardly called me into the conversations all evening and everyone got to see how skilled he's going to be at Charades! Many thanks to all involved for your great ideas and work to make this weekend happen for us! After a great breakfast together Sunday, we had a peaceful drive home, stopping at Buckhead Ridge to look for the old Gator Den (Hutcherson family's fish camp), but much has changed since we had been there five years ago and it's nowhere to be found.

This past weekend was a short visit with Kim and Kevin who are doing well as empty-nesters and in the throes of retirement planning and downsizing; always good to be with them. Then Dale and I watched lots of volleyball at U of Tampa camp where Christy had three teams competing. Although this Gulf Coast HS is a young, they look real good and it was great to see how the younger players fit right in. UT coach Chris Catanach reminded us that he and Dale have known each other since 1985, Chris's first year at UT when he hosted US Olympic setter Debbie Green at his first camp. Dale had taken his volleyball teams to UT camp annually and now Christy is doing the same. And our daughter Lin played volleyball for Chris her sophomore year in college. We SO enjoyed reconnecting with the volleyball girls; it was Dale's first time since October.

We are settled comfortably into short weeks at home. This week, we'll have our last day watching all three grandsons at golf camp and Dale will have his first opportunity to hit tennis balls with a longtime coaching friend. Speech sessions are twice a week now and Dale is no longer imitating teacher's sounds, but generating sounds, words, and short sentences on his own. His conversational actions (eye contact, waiting on other's responses, etc.) have become normal and we see regular improvement in speech. Frustration and impatience still surface for both of us several times a week, but God is faithful to remind us of the positive and show us the next step to take as we encourage one another.

Family is still a major source of support and encouragement, whether in person or by phone, and friends are tremendously important to us as well. Thank you for your prayers and love, a never-ending source of strength for us. We postponed GA mountain hiking plans once we realized that wisdom would dictate we hike desolate places with others, not alone, so we'll wait for the right time that others can join us. Any takers? We're off to Gainesville this weekend and then will spend a few days in Tallahassee with family.

7/21/2015 Neurofatigue... Unseen Consequences of Brain Injury

FYI - very real and very important. Here's a link with a good explanation:

https://www.braininjury-explanation.com/consequences/invisible-consequences/neurofatigue

Scan here for more information

Friends with an injured brain state they cannot handle multiple sensory input like radio <u>and</u> GPS in the car; it results in sensory overload. Few people understand what it means to describe your brain as *tired*. It is something that has to be experienced or discussed *in depth* with one going through it and can sometimes occur simply when typical aspects of life become exhausting in and of themselves. Although this is so very real to the individual with TBI, it can be very difficult for others to grasp. Patience and understanding are key, along with not treating it the same as physical exhaustion.

8/11/2015 Six Months Home

August 1st marked six months that Dale's been home from rehab and ten months since the stroke. We continue to move forward. Our pace is often not what we'd like, but patience is a fruit of the Spirit, and we see evidence of that building in our lives. Trials do that; God is faithful, and we trust Him. It is not easy for me to put myself in Dale's shoes, not being able to communicate. Most of the time he handles it with persistence, but frustration bubbles up and we have then to figure a way to resolve the situation at hand. Tears have been fewer, but we're not holding back. Some lonely times, too, but those cause me to listen to God and often end in reaching out to others.

Our Gainesville trip was definitely a success. We spent Friday night to Sunday noon watching Christy's Gulf Coast HS volleyball team in all their competitions. Dale was in his element and loved it! He had a few communications with Christy about players and got to reconnect with a number of the GCHS volleyball family. It was heartwarming. They had been SO supportive of us and Christy during the worst times. Staying on campus provided us with short walks to the venues when weather permitted; UF is still a special place to us both. Visits with the local friends were a highlight as well, friendships that have spanned many decades. Thank you, Lord. Then we enjoyed the drive to Tallahassee, a few days with all of Carol's family and relaxing times at their wooded property.

I'm recently realizing that Dale is directing his own therapy more and more, rebuffing many of my suggestions; I've had to surrender this to God, knowing that He is directing and in control, not me, and that my role is continually changing as Dale recovers. God's design of the brain is more than we'll ever comprehend. I'm just grateful for all the recent knowledge that has been revealed through research and is an encouragement to us. Dale's therapy now is through skills and activities such as exercise, gym workouts, cooking breakfast, and typical household chores. It's easy to take things for granted; we do well to remember how these were a struggle only six months ago—shaving, using the remote, sorting clothes, and using the gym equipment without assistance. Gradual, successful, consistent improvement is still happening; speech takes the most effort.

Dale has had three tennis sessions with a friend/coach that have been encouraging; he shows progress in tracking the ball, and that always remind us that the reconnections are happening. We can see familiar movements in his forehand and backhand that simply need fine tuning. Of course, the fine tuning takes detailed instruction that he manages best in baby steps right now. Guitar sessions have been going on for a month, once a week with a friend from church who doesn't claim to be a teacher but is a gift from God and works/relates well with Dale. Last session, Dale played the first two lines from

Only in God (John Michael Talbot) consistently correct; they've been working on that for three weeks. He feels good about these sessions. They are definitely his interests and very therapeutic. We often notice that as improvement comes in one area, other actions progress as well over the next few days.

"All boats float on a rising tide."

For a week now, since our weekend travels finished, we've been on a juice fast for cleansing and health. Prepared for a week by reducing caffeine and adding fresh juice daily so the transition has been far better than I expected. I'm strictly on juice; Dale has eggs, meat, or nuts as he feels the need. I've encouraged him to do as he is led. I do the juicing and he fixes anything else. Will reassess weekly.

> *God's design of the brain is more than we'll ever comprehend. I'm just grateful for all the recent knowledge that has been revealed through research and is an encouragement to us.*

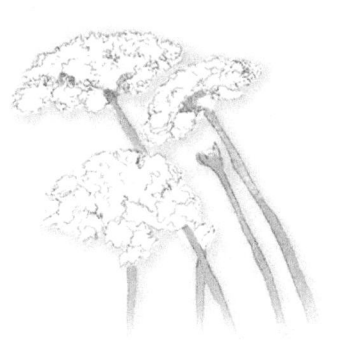

The friend who's been living with us while in job transition has a week's vacation August 18-24 and will be traveling to Ohio and back; that presented us with an unforeseen opportunity to drive up with him. His home is an hour from Pittsburgh where Dale's speech therapist lives. So, he can drop us off in Pittsburgh and Dale is scheduled to have morning and afternoon face-to-face SLP sessions. Very exciting! Our plans are simple. We are staying downtown and won't need a car. It will be the longest trip we've had, and we will stop overnight near Charlotte, NC. I have to pack for a week (it will take me a week to do that, having much to consider circumspectly).

And we were blessed with God's provision of finances from outside sources to be devoted to Dale's therapy before this trip came about. Isn't that like God? We just didn't know the future! In addition, we get to see a Pirates game at PNC park, adding to my growing list of baseball parks visited over the years. (Yes, I happen to be a baseball fan, raised in the 50's listening on my transistor to the Yankees in the World Series during elementary school!)

We are trusting God and walking through doors He opens. Someone approached us last week to work with Dale on art therapy for an hour a week and we look forward to how that impacts his continued recovery. We are grateful for each person who prays, offers help, visits, or meets any need we have; we know we are not in this alone. Thanks to each of you; when you reach out to us, the impact is noticeable, and your prayers are felt.

8/17/2015 – Daily Doings

These are times of growth and interaction. I'm personally glad to be back on the porch as lower night temps were most welcome and some grayer afternoons or cooling rains brought low 80s in the pre-dinner hours. This river view is solace and refreshing that brings deep satisfaction, especially for me.

I need You, Lord, in the daily doings, the tedious tasks, and the patient planning. Every moment of every day, I need You. Thank you, Holy Spirit, for Your guidance, presence, wisdom, and love. You are my everything and I praise You. Even in that I need you; my every breath. Without You, I can do *nothing*.

8/31/15 Pittsburgh Visit

I expected to review this trip as soon as we got back, but it's taken a week for me to carve out enough time to do it justice. What a blessing to have this opportunity! After a l-o-n-g drive, we arrived

Wednesday afternoon and found the Wyndham to be all we had hoped. It was comfortable, centrally located on the triangle, and had a nice view of the city. After meeting Dale's speech therapist in a brief face-to-face introduction, we walked the city streets and dined at Meat & Potatoes on possibly the best lamb steak we've had, while surrounded by diners enjoying marrow from LARGE bones, which was a new sight for us to see.

Thursday, our SLP picked us up at 9:00 a.m. and, as a Pittsburgh native, provided us with running commentary on his city during the ten-minute drive to his office where we met other Speech Language Pathologists (SLPs) who we came to know and appreciate. The morning was spent with much Q&A evaluation, making the most of the "in person" meeting time (previous to now, sessions had been via WebEx video conferencing since January). We spent our lunch break outside at old Market Square, enjoying beautiful weather, a farmer's market, and PPG's great architecture (a favorite of mine). Afternoon brought more evaluations, then more intense speech sessions. Around 4:00 p.m. after a tenuous time of feeling "graded," Dale had an emotional meltdown. After a walk and conversation outside, he asked me to voice his concerns, understandably based on weariness and fears. Those were addressed by the director in a rational, professional manner, stating some of his business tenets, including having no planned discharge date from therapy; *discharge here is based on the client's recognition of reaching their goals and discharging the therapists, rather than vice-versa.* He firmly stated that whenever the therapists were stymied, it was THEIR JOB to work to find solutions. With Dale's concerns resolved, we were able to move forward in a positive atmosphere of trust.

We were then treated to a short tour of the building where the therapy is housed - the historic Pittsburgh Brewery (still functioning on the lower level), and to an excellent Italian meal at the old Legends restaurant on the north side. Dale and his SLP have had a wonderful relationship over the past eight months. They are around the same age and have much in common in athletics and coaching. With my description of Dale now being a "language athlete" in rehab, all the SLPs now capitalize on Dale's knowledge and experience of coaching techniques, years of teaching Anatomy and AP Bio, and understanding of the needs of rehabilitation. It's been a blessing.

Friday morning, an associate picked us up on her way to the office, having stopped first at Antney's to bring us her favorite homemade ice cream in a cooler! Thursday she uncovered Dale's love of ice cream and mentioned this amazing ice cream place with unique flavors – we were hooked. We decided on ice cream for breakfast and enjoyed every bite - refreshing and fun!

In the morning session, everyone had to state one word describing yesterday—change, perplexing, relaxing, insightful, challenging—and we composed a sentence that incorporated goals along with humor. *"Calm change in a relaxed manner will sure as heck allow insight into Dale's perplexing challenge!"*

Comfortable conversation encouraged all of us, and Dale thrived in this atmosphere. Clarification was stated that speech was not the foremost challenge, that Dale *had* the words and needed to speak with confidence, talk more, and let it flow. Cognition will be the major emphasis, attacking apraxia at every turn ("Apraxia affects motor speech production. This means that if someone with aphasia can think of the words they want to say, the part of their brain that coordinates the movements to say those words gets a fuzzy signal or no signal at all.")[3] One SLP worked on association, another on semantics, building more ways to communicate what Dale wants to say. Lunch was at Habitat in the Fairmont Hotel specializing in local,

---

[3] (The Aphasia Center n.d.)

seasonal fare; we feasted on Chilled Fresh Pea Soup, Spinach Salad with grilled peaches, pine nuts, berries and creme fraiche, and Wild Arugula Salad with braised duck and watermelon. Bon Appetit!

In the afternoon, pragmatics of conversation were outlined and practiced such as eye contact, speaking with confidence and projecting, exhibiting clear gestures when confused or needing a restart, taking time to think, processing his thoughts and speech, and giving time for the other party to verify/confirm what Dale said. What an awesome help! Having taught speech to high schoolers, most of these were familiar to me, but having the "expert" direct this with Dale gave us powerful tools for communication, which were implemented from that time forward. Our day ended with a walk across Roberto Clemente bridge to see a Pirates game vs Giants at PNC Park from third-tier third base seats overlooking the city skyline as the sun set. It was perfect!

Saturday morning, we met Dale's SLP at Gold's Gym for a workout, then to Market Square for coffee and scones at Nicholas' Coffee Company (est.1920) where they still roast coffee beans and grind fresh peanut butter—my kind of place! After another intensive speech session, our tour of the city continued on a drive leading us to the Carnegie Museum of Natural History and Art Museum. We could have spent the whole day there, but filled up our two hours with Dale's favorites being the paleontology lab and the dinosaur displays (ranked #4 in the US) and my favorite area of gems and minerals. The tour continued past colleges, through streets of old mansions, and along the river, ending at our hotel. More strolling through the city, ogling at the PPG brilliant architecture, and dining sumptuously at Il Pizzaiolo on our now favorite Market Square.

Packed and ready to leave on Sunday morning, we spent our final Sunday morning hours at the Fort Pitt Museum and Point State Park on the riverfront. After a smooth and uneventful eighteen-hour drive home, Dale has been reignited to engage in as many therapies as possible, fueled by the knowledge that his brain reconnections improve with any area that moves forward.

Counting our blessings:
- being included in our houseguest's vacation drive home, easy travel, good company
- financial provision for this trip
- good music and historical audiobooks that we all enjoyed
- great accommodations and beautiful walking weather
- innovative, caring therapists with personalized care during our visit
- Pittsburgh, a new city to love, and great tickets for the Pirates' game
- further knowledge to help Dale's continued recovery

9/19/2015 Go Gators!

With no real apologies to those who are not Gator or football fans, this journal entry bleeds of **orange** and **blue**! Dale played for one of the best Florida teams to ever set foot in the Swamp, the 1969 Gators, and these guys have remained in touch throughout the years. This past weekend, their coach, Ray Graves, was honored before the game and Dale joined so many of the guys from the 'Silver Sixties' gathered in Coach's memory; they got to be on the field together, forming a tunnel for this year's team as they entered before 90,000 cheering fans. Brought back some great memories!

We also enjoyed time together, wonderful fellowship, that afternoon at a gathering with delicious authentic Cuban food. Dale interacted very comfortably with the fifty or so players and families from the '69 team who welcomed and embraced him. It was encouraging for him and heartwarming for me to have these friends engage him in conversation as well as guide him onto the field (and back!).

The game was a blast as the team led by a new coaching staff romped over the opponent 61-13! From our seats we had a great view of the south endzone where at least half of the touchdowns took place... as well as the fireworks from the top of the jumbotron. Christy and our three "adopted" daughters sat with us along with Gator friends. Weather was perfect and cool, and we spent halftime in F Club to greet a longtime friend and get a bite to eat. A truly great day!

It is continually evident to us that we are blessed to grow old with our friends and that relationships grow richer with the years. These guys included three of the groomsmen from our wedding and some families we've known since college. In addition, Friday night dinner was with our dear family friends; always a precious time. Many thanks to all who made this event possible... **Go Gators!**

9/27/2015 It's the Little Things...

A listening ear, a phone call, a hand on your shoulder, or a small, unexpected gift often bring just the encouragement needed to face the next hour, the next phone call, the next step. We've been the grateful recipients of these for nearly a year and are just as blessed to be able to encourage others.

This week, we attended a stroke support group, something that was never in *our* plans but God had our attention when Dale's former OT saw us this week for the first time since April on our regular workout visit to the Y. She noticed us from the rehab adjacent to the gym entrance and actually came running out to greet us and hand us a flyer, encouraging us to attend this group that she was leading, saying she'd been wanting to reach us, but Dale's info was no longer in their system. We trust her, so I looked at the first meeting date and realized it was **in thirty minutes right at that location, and we were already there**! Thanks, God. We know to trust Him in all circumstances and that this was not coincidental, so we adjusted our workouts and went in with a good attitude, acknowledging that this could be an opportunity both to learn and to help someone else. We listened to everyone's story and were able to give some feedback and encouragement. The "lineup" for speakers through May sounds as though we may gain some further knowledge. Opportunities to relate to others were most evident right from the start—a Gator fan, someone who gained from us sharing our personal card, receiving encouragement from others' positive outlooks, and encouraging others to find their place in these new relationships. I volunteered to give resource reviews, mostly of books, and am scheduled to speak at the December meeting. Dale's OT gave me a new book to read; I've finished it, gaining new insights already this week!

Grateful to be of help to others, we will walk through doors that open for us and hope to bring encouragement in any area. We all need it. By the time some of you read this, it will be a year since Dale had the stroke on October 3rd. Please keep us in prayer, especially that evening, as I've already been engaged in battle with the enemy and have had to look fear in the face, knowing that God is greater and His love casts out all fear. We will celebrate Dale's continuing life and the victory we've both had during his recovery time. His 65th birthday is October 9th and we'll have dinner with the family.

The little things... this week we were able to get to Siesta Beach for a walk on a beautiful day. It's one of our favorite places and just a simple walk on the beach brought such blessing; we are so glad to have this beach nearby. Your simple prayer as you read this, and words of encouragement, truly mean so much. We know that everyone has much going on in their own lives and we thank you for all your efforts on our behalf.

There is still much to be done and the therapies continue such as speech, cognition/perception, physical hand/eye coordination through art, and sports and guitar. Dale still has speech three times a week and each of the others once a week, with additional practice as he can fit it in. It all fills our days along with workouts and time outdoors and with family; evenings remain relaxed (except for that last Gator win over Tennessee!).

9/28/2015 Energy is Key

I'm reflecting on neurofatigue after Dale had a couple of sub-par days. There's still SO much to learn even though we've all been learning so much. Energy is key. We have seen much recovery and are living life as fully as Dale is able, yet the energy drain on Dale's brain is affected by EVERY stimulation—positive or negative—and his energy gets sapped so much more quickly, and sometimes suddenly. Everything he does and we do affects his energy, even if it's emotionally positive. This is the number one aftereffect of the stroke, and I again reference the manual/automatic car transmission analogy. He definitely moves in manual transmission, and it requires much more energy than when everything was on automatic. Additionally, he can neither express it nor grasp the concept of what is happening and why unless we discuss it in the moment. Hard changes for us both; actually, for the entire family.

I told David last night that since Dad is so greatly affected energy-wise by many factors such as focus, new environment/people, intensity, and emotion that we can no longer consider the family trip to Europe that we had hoped for once we both were retired. So, Lord, I lay that before You, our different life, doing what we can and recognizing what we shouldn't do. Lead on. This isn't about me or about Europe, but about Your plan for us all. I am at peace with Your plans, content to follow You, and rest in Your care. Thank You for Your loving guidance:

<u>G</u>od <u>U</u> + *I* <u>D A N C E</u>.   Lead on!

Chapter Seven

MARKING ONE YEAR

10/6/15 Just Being Real... One Year Later

What a difference a year makes! None of us are the same people we were a year ago. Noteworthy for us **this** year is that we have specific markers by which we can measure or gauge our changes. That is interesting, if not welcome.

October 3rd marked a year since Dale's stroke and this past week has provoked much reflection with both thankfulness and regret. Both of us have had to face the truth that we are not where we ever expected to be nor where we hoped to be and that our personal situation has produced significant changes in every aspect of our lives. That being said, Dale has times that memories surface and need to be dealt with in the moment; his rational thinking is nowhere near what it was prior to the stroke, and I am grateful when it does come into play. Reflection and evaluation on my part is a daily occurrence as I note changes and shift the flow of our daily lives to incorporate them and respond accordingly, thankful for the guidance of Holy Spirit to give me mindfulness as He leads. God directs what each of us can handle and we cast our cares on Him; that is not a platitude for us, but a way of living in the present and purposing to only bear our part. I have had a conscious giving over of cares to Father; Dale is graced by Him for this time with the freedom to not have an understanding of the many possible cares, and in that we both are blessed.

Considering growth/change over the years, we would turn to Luke 2:52 *"And Jesus grew in <u>wisdom</u> and <u>stature</u>, and in <u>favor with God</u> and <u>men</u>,"* so I naturally evaluate this year's growth in those areas:

-<u>Wisdom</u> (knowledge, mental and emotional growth) - Volumes of knowledge - brain, medical care, trauma, recovery; about ourselves - how we respond to challenge, pain, heartbreak...
-<u>Stature</u> (the physical) - Details of how the body works, grows, changes, heals, rests; nutritional intake, energy output; the learning and retraining process...
-<u>Favor with God</u> (spiritual) - Father's love and faithfulness; that He is our Rock, our Hope, our Wisdom, our Strength, our All in All, a very present Help in time of need; that we can trust Him implicitly and continually know Him more; He has Divine appointments for us with so many individuals just right for the moment...
-<u>Favor with men</u> (social) - the ups/downs, joys/pains of human relationships, the amazing, helpful responses of so many and, conversely, the loneliness experienced by being "different" ...

In the midst of all events, circumstances, medical tests and care, rehab, recovery, prayers, well wishes, tears, laughter, visits, and travels, **this is what we KNOW:**
>-God always surrounded us, going before and behind us; His Presence evident in circumstances and direction
>-people and places came into our lives to minister for specific needs, some only seen for the moment and never again
>-resources continue to surface and we continue to learn
>-the brain is always changing; change is growth and continues when stimulated
>-fear is not of God and peace happens in the midst of chaos
>-God has a plan for our lives and it continues

Growing... changing... moving forward... following His plan... we are blessed.

10/22/2015 Ordinary Life

OR-DI-NAR-Y adjective: *customary, normal, standard, typical, common, usual, habitual, everyday, regular, routine, day-to-day*

This will be the last of any regular entries; our life now has more ordinary elements than extraordinary. That being said, we still live "out of the ordinary," aware of the uniqueness of days, moments, interactions, and the gift of each day being special in and of itself. We have opportunity to be fully alive every day we're alive.

We have settled into the common (for us), the "new normal" which in itself changes day by day yet has these customary elements:
- sleep/wake schedule with Dale still on sleep medication
- brain-healthy diet 90+% of the time
- a variety of therapies, emphasis on speech/communication
- continual awareness of Dale's energy level/neurofatigue
- wind down after 7:00 p.m.
- social interaction, visits, and travel
- appropriate physical activity and conditioning
- fresh air, sunshine, and appreciation for nature
- independent living activities for Dale, continuing to increase
- reading and audiobooks; conscious learning
- spiritual growth and prayer
- family time
- time apart from each other for mental rest, even in snatches
- "living life" and appreciating the freedom of retirement

Those of you who have read this journal, kept in touch, prayed for us, and encouraged us both are a highly important and effective part of Dale's recovery and my sanity. Please continue to interact with us as you can, including visits. The guest room is ready and waiting, the pool is inviting, and the view from the porch is restorative.

> *"The Lord bless you and keep you;*
> *The Lord make His face shine upon you,*
> *And be gracious to you;*
> *The Lord lift up His countenance upon you,*
> *And give you peace."*
> *Numbers 6:24-26*

11/8/2015 Change Your Brain, Change Your Life

We want to share this wonderful in brain information with you. We have learned much from Dr. Daniel Amen since 2006 (*pre-stroke*) and have implemented much of his wisdom, more intently since Dale stroked. In the link below, Amen lists twelve prescriptions to optimize your brain. *We highly recommend **everyone** read this, no matter your age.* There has been an amazing research on the brain in the past ten years, bringing much info into the public realm; we all benefit from learning about and caring for our magnificent brains.

https://www.danielplan.com/-change-your-brain-change-your-life/

Scan here for more information

11/16/2015 Reflections On Pine Mountain Trip

I do rejoice in You, Lord, and trust You. When darkness and fear come upon me, Your Truth rises, and Your counsel sets me free. Without You, we can do NOTHING, so I run to You, put my hope and trust in You. I want to live in You, walk continually with You, serve You alone, my Rock and my Strength.

Lead on, Lord. This trip to Pine Mountain served for rest and reflection, not as I saw it, but as You planned it.

We met Kim and Kevin for a Gator game with great anticipation. Overall, a good day, however, we sat in full sun, and it did a number on Dale's energy. When I realized he was overheating, it took a good deal of maneuvering to get him through the crowd to shade and a cooling drink/ice. (One of the first recognitions of his major lack of self-evaluating.) We were on an upper level and to get him downstairs, they allowed us to use the elevator, but he passed out on the way down. I had help in getting him to the First Aid area, then the F Club with AC and good care, but felt he needed to rest/recover and not drive two hours to Carol's in Tallahassee. Friends in town came to the rescue and after a good night's sleep, Dale had recovered, and we were on our way. Once in Pine Mountain, the facilities were wonderful, but I was FULLY aware that I needed caution in all we attempted as I was really on my own for care should anything happen. It was a place of rest and enjoyment, and I had much time to reflect and consider the newness of encountering familiar circumstances with unfamiliar life changes:

-reality of Dale's energy and pace
-my role in that
-consideration from his viewpoint
-seeking wise counsel
-God bringing counsel forth
-encouragement

Thank You for good friends and visits, cool weather, beautiful scenery, peaceful places, deer, chipmunks, ladybugs, good food, comfortable beds, and rest.

NOTE: In retrospect, it is likely that Dale had an AFib episode at the game and possibly slighter episodes the end of September, not understood or noted by him but highly affecting his energy. It was not detected as the medics at the stadium checked him after he passed out. However, important new medical evidence about Dale's condition would soon come to light, as revealed in the next few Caring Bridge entries, dated just two weeks later.

Chapter Eight

STROKED AGAIN – RESET THE REHAB CLOCK

12/3/15 Stroked Again

Although I'm grateful to be in the familiar surroundings of Sarasota Memorial, this is not where we had hoped to be. Yesterday, Dale had a stroke in the posterior cerebellum and was admitted to Sarasota Memorial Neuro ICU last night after going to the ER in North Port. There is no paralysis, gratefully, but his vision is quite impaired with a lot of neglect (meaning he has limitations/neglect in his field of vision—homonymous hemianopsia, see photo from 10/10/14), basically because of the location of the stroke. His comprehension is excellent, but his following of instructions is very confused. We have met with doctors, have a great neurologist, and they are rechecking all Dale's cardiology tests to see if they can find a cause. His vitals stabilized overnight; he is not on any medication except anticoagulants and can have Tylenol if there's a headache. He's on normal food and is swallowing well (although he presently needs assistance with eating due to the sight issues). I'm very pleased with the doctors and they are happy that all his records are in their system for review. That sure gives more credence to what I've been sharing with them! He should spend most of the day sleeping as he was up late last night and there's a lot of bells and whistles here. Hopefully he'll be moved from there once evaluations are finished.

I am well, just need more sleep. I have been exercising in Dale's room doing squats, wall pushups, and stretches. I have a better handle on needs since last year's experiences—Dale's and mine.

David, Christy, and other trusted counsel are in place, two siblings and spouses live in Sarasota, and my other two sisters are on call to come as needed. God is providing and I am grateful. SO thankful this didn't happen on our Pine Mountain trip.

12/4/15 Good Rest

Good morning! Dale is still sleeping, so I'm down in the courtyard having breakfast. Yesterday, he was evaluated by all the therapists, and I got to meet with his main doctor/neurologist, and the cardiologist. They're still for the cause of the blood clot and will do a procedure today to track his heart rhythm and check for A-fib. Very good care here, and they are listening both to my concerns and questions and honoring our desire for no statins or opiates.

We've kept the room as quiet as possible and are keeping additional stimulation to a minimum so he can rest and heal. Although vision is impaired on the left side and depth perception is off, by evening Dale showed big improvements after a day of rest. He sat in the chair twice for over an hour, walked around the unit with assistance, and ate a lot of his dinner by himself, even finding chicken and broccoli with his fork and finding and picking up his drinks by himself. He's waiting to go for another walk before settling down.

This morning's report is that he had a good and quiet night, only getting up for the bathroom which is typical. Had his meds at 8:00 p.m. so this gives him good, long rest. I'm thankful and am not surprised by the quality and duration of sleep with his "normal" sleep medication that he's been using for a year.

Today he has that procedure at 1:00 p.m. Kevin is hoping to stop by for a visit before that, and we hope to see three friends who are working here today. That should make a full day.

12/5/15 Good Report and "My Best Friend Has a Saying..."

Therapy activities prevented me from writing earlier, so here's yesterday's recap. Day went slowly as Dale had to fast until one, so he rested most of the morning. His procedure to insert a 'loop' to monitor heart rhythm went well and then he was discharged from SMH and moved to CRU, the Comprehensive Rehab Unit encased on a floor right within the hospital. We met with the directing doctor, who was very well-versed on Dale's case history, and conversed with each of us thoroughly. Unfortunately, making a major change in venue late in the day left no opportunity to acclimate to surroundings and with shift change at 7:00 p.m., we had to meet two sets of staff within an hour. Dale was then very anxious about the new place; bad memories flooded in and he had to battle fear. I decided to stay the night and was welcomed to use the empty bed. Niece Michelle and friend came for a short visit and were a good diversion. We got Dale to laugh at the end telling a joke. A family friend, a nurse at SMH, was the angel God sent at the perfect time to assure us both that we're in the best place; she worked on this floor for over two years and knows most of the staff. God is good. Dale got night meds early at 7:00 p.m. and he slept well, unlike me....

Today Dale is stable and well-rested after twelve hours sleep, but sad early this morning. Breakfasted in dining room, fed himself, and met some other patients; all meals are in dining room. Had OT at 9:00 a.m. and did great with washing, dressing, etc. Hemianopsia vision is classic - down the middle with no field of vision on the left, but the neglect has basically disappeared as he compensates by turning his head, sometimes needing to be cued to "look around" to find what he's looking for. Speech therapy was wonderful with a gal we had met last year; his speech has recovered back to what is normal for him. Hallelujah! He then passed PT with flying colors and only needs someone to walk nearby because of what he might miss due to vision cuts. We expect by Tuesday when the director returns, they will be able to give us realistic plan to return home.

I got four to five hours of sleep, and we both napped about an hour this afternoon. I will be going back to my friends' tonight as staff is doing all they can to assist and I saw Dale's ability to deal with bed alarm during the night, plus they will leave a light on for him.

Thank you for your prayers; they especially carry us through times when we are tired, and our weaknesses are evident. May God continue to show Himself strong during those times.

I'll end with this: the unit's director asked Dale if he had questions when our conversation was ending. Dale said, "Why? I'm scared. Will it happen again?" They were very real and emotional questions that we all have. Doctor said, *"My best friend has a saying 'Don't worry about tomorrow; tomorrow will worry about itself. Each day has enough trouble of its own.'"* I said, "Well, our best friend is Jesus, and He tells us that," to which he said, "That's the friend I meant and in all the times I've shared that, you're the first to ever identify it." What a blessing to be under the ministry of this man!

12/6/15 Bittersweet

Today, we found out that Dale has Atrial Fibrillation (AFib) which very well may be the source of blood clots/stroke. Last year in searching for the cause of Dale's stroke, thorough testing was done including every cardiac test; no problems were found. This week Dale already had a TEE and an echocardiogram; both showed no irregularities. This morning, Dale had two odd weak spells, one at breakfast with pain near the incision site on his chest, and one after sitting for a while then standing up. His nurses were wise enough to check his vitals, found his blood pressure was low, called the cardiologist, and ordered an EKG which showed AFib. We were immediately grateful to be closer to identifying a cause of his strokes. He was prescribed Eliquis, a blood thinner which has no vitamin K restrictions as Coumadin does. Started that today along with Metoprolol, a beta blocker to regulate his heartbeat. Blood work was done to be checked for troponin increase, a protein that would indicate if any damage was done to his heart.

Dale's activity level was noticeably affected throughout the day and that was emotional for me to watch, along with the recognition that he now has to be on two medications. We are thankful for these effective medications and the positive outcome they should have on Dale's body. Please pray for adjustment to his system. Dale's lower energy levels today affected his cognition by late afternoon, usually hard for me as he tends to experience more confusion and/or agitation. Please pray for that whole aspect of his recovery. Winding down is always more difficult away from home; presently it's still affected by vision issues and as his energy is waning more quickly, his need to wind down occurs earlier in the day. Overall, we certainly are counting our blessings and are thankful for:
- AFib surfacing while Dale was hospitalized good care
- Dale remaining positive all day and being at peace with this new knowledge and medication, even when he was tired
- his acclimation to and trust in the CRU staff
- peace when I leave at night and good rest for both of us
- wise, experienced, caring medical staff
- God's encouragement to us through so many various people
- our dear friend's love and hospitality

12/7/15 Adjusting

A good night's sleep for both of us, even with Dale gaining a roommate. Dale had a good day overall; his BP was still a little low this morning so he was required to have someone near him whenever he walked around. Noticeably stronger than yesterday, did well at therapies and passed shower evaluation. We went outside to the courtyard for a while - a beautiful day to be in the fresh air. Seems like the meds are doing what they should, and I continue to tell him that his job is 1) to rest so he can heal and 2) to work hard in rehab so he can go home. We'll learn more from his rehab team Thursday.

Please pray for insight/wisdom concerning meds, and careful consideration from the doctors concerning the long term use of Seroquel and other possible sleep aids, all of which I am prayerfully considering. I hope to see all the doctors in next day or so.

Thank you all for your encouragement and suggestions. Days are long and there is not much to do here; it wears on both of us and is sometimes quite a struggle for me to creatively initiate things to do. Always looking for ideas; listening to Christmas music today!

12/9/2015 Great News!

Coming home tomorrow morning! More info later.

12/10/15 All Roads Lead to Home

Thank you, Lord! We are ever so grateful to be going home and for all that God has done since we were at SMH. We are witness to the truth that *"all things work together for good for those who love Him and are called according to His purpose"* (Romans 8:28). In the midst of life's storms, God's faithfulness has always shone through. We give Him glory and proclaim these blessings from this week:
    -excellent care and caring staff
    -doctors who listened and were thorough in their considerations and explanations
    -the MANY prayers offered on our behalf
    -family, friends who were able to visit
    -our friend's precious friendship and hospitality
    -Dale has a cardiologist and neurologist (previously needed)
    -a cause for strokes was found and solutions administered

-a plan to wean off night meds with help of a sleep specialist
-our home served as a friend's haven while we were gone
-the CRU piano gave us opportunity to sing a few mornings, joined by others; also Christmas carols at lunch Wednesday
-met Gator fans
-connected with a volleyball player who had played against Christy in HS (and her father was Donna's HS teacher!)
-had beautiful weather to enjoy outside in the courtyards
-CRU dining room has the best hospital view of Sarasota Bay

That being said, there's no place like HOME!!

12/11/15 Desired Haven

We are grateful to be home; I'm including truth from God's Word that speaks directly to our present situation.

Psalm 107:28-30: *Then they cried to the LORD in their trouble, and he delivered them from their distress. He made the storm be still, and the waves of the sea were hushed. Then they were GLAD that the waters were quiet, and he brought them to their DESIRED HAVEN. Let them give thanks to the Lord for His unfailing love and His wonderful deeds for mankind.*

This is our first full day home. I'm not sure why this scripture came to mind as I sat down to write, but I do know that we are involved in spiritual battle. It is evident that Dale needs rest; he slept twelve hours last night, and now, twelve hours later, he's back in bed – down for the night. Having said that, we were going to rest this weekend, that in itself is a challenge, and yet we both need it in abundance. Fortunately, Dale is not anxious to do anything in particular and is not mindful of all that "needs" to be done. That is good. He sang with me at the piano this morning, visited with the neighbor, walked around the property here, and watched a movie; he went down for a nap, but didn't sleep. That's when fears and questions began to surface in his mind, so we rested next to each other and talk quietly about Truth. *"You shall know the truth and the truth shall set you free"* John 8:32. Fear has no place in this house or in us; for decades we have loved and lived by Psalm 3:5-6 *"Trust in the Lord with all your heart and lean not to your own understanding; in all your ways acknowledge Him, and He will direct your paths."* Step by step... we really only need to see what next steps we should take, not all the way to the end of the road, and we CAN trust that His Word lights our path (Psalm 119:105)

For the many of you that remind me to take care of myself, I did sleep well last night and I appreciate your reminders and assistance. I am very conscious of all that needs to be done; my personal challenge is not just to be doing, but to be listening to what I am to do. Food prep was already done for a few days and I'm keeping it simple; laundry got done today along with phone calls for follow-up doctor visits. I'm glad to have those things off my list and my mind. I am looking forward to what comes next and to creating an atmosphere for healing and restoration.

> *Step by step... we really only need to see what next steps we should take, not all the way to the end of the road, and we CAN trust that His Word lights our path. (Psalm 119:105)*

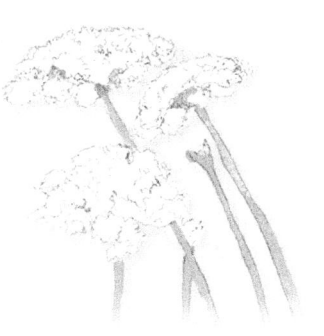

Conversing and repeating everything is tiring; thank you for understanding and realizing that I don't have much down time, and by the time I do, I'd rather be still. I am thankful for the gift of technology although I count it a blessing and a curse. Right now, journaling here serves me well to reflect and ruminate (yes, like a cow - no comments, please) and have the opportunity to update and, hopefully, encourage family and friends.

Thank you for caring enough to keep up with us and thank you for praying; we are relying on it because we can't do this alone.

12/12/2015 Best Advice Today

From a kindhearted Gator friend: "**Get your rest, turn off the world, and live YOUR life.**" Thank you, Lord, for compassionate, insightful souls. I *do* rest in You.

12/15/15 So Glad to be Home – Englewood

We moved back to Englewood three years ago after Dale retired (for the second time), and we have been extraordinarily blessed by settling back into this hometown. I remember when we moved here in 1979 how we truly felt led here by God to be planted here and raise our family. The history we have within this community is rich, from buying our first home on the very first day we came down (and sold our previous home the same day!), to adding another daughter to our family, to the twenty-four years Dale taught/coached at Lemon Bay HS and the stories that unfold after decades of investing in the people of this community. Rich... rewarding... rooted, a perfect fit for this 3rd generation Floridian and his coastal-loving wife. Even with having moved away for ten years, this is HOME. As we've maneuvered along new paths in the past year, so much encouragement has come from the landmark relationships we've had in this wonderful laid-back town.

That fact was evidenced again yesterday as we visited our primary care doctor for Dale's follow-up. He and we are knit into the fabric of this community and our lives have been interwoven - his dad was our doctor for years and both of us having taught/coached his brother. It was comforting and rich to have a health conversation with both him and his nurse having history with us. We are blessed, and for me to be in this new position of decision-making for the both of us, I relish this honest and heartfelt counsel on which to rely. Definitely God planned through the years for a time such as this; our entire family benefits from this history. Thank you, Lord.

This brief account barely touches the surface of all the blessings that we have from being in this community, including the home we built for our family and the place where we are now living on the Myakka River; blessings we count daily. In addition, the medical team that has been put together for Dale's health is amazing and includes doctors from Sarasota that our Englewood doctor knows and honors. Consequently, our many questions have been answered, and our knowledge and direction of how to address Dale's health needs continues to move forward, fine tuning his care.

Today, we visited the cardiologist; Thursday, Dale will be evaluated by OT and Speech for outpatient rehab; next week is the neurologist visit. A sleep doctor is now part of this team to hopefully wean Dale off pharmaceuticals while still maintaining good sleep so he can continue to heal. And today, to complete Dale's team, we heard from the neuropsychologist referred by our PCP and will meet after the first of the year. Although it may be more doctors than many would want, for us these and therapists are an answer to prayer, evaluating and directing our walk toward Dale's complete restoration.

Many of you have been praying with us to that end and we want you to be encouraged by all that has happened since Dale suffered this recent stroke:
- -AFib discovered to be the source of the blood clots and medicines prescribed that work to resolve the issue and are in concert with our personal health lifestyle
- -incorporating wonderful doctors into Dale's team

-evaluations and input from therapists that brought new perspectives and possibilities
-longtime friends are now available for a time to assist us with therapies and daily living
-a "reset" for our daily schedule with fresh eyes on how to wisely spend our hours
-addressing fear head-on and giving it NO place in our lives

Please be praying for us about each of these things this week as we hope to establish a routine that gives Dale a variety of therapies, moves him to independent daily living, gives us flexibility to interact with others socially, and grows us both to serve God and others.

May God's peace overwhelm you and give you true rest this weekend.

12/17/15 It's The Little Things...

So, I have "needed" two boxes for odd-sized Christmas gifts. I really appreciate being able to wrap gifts so what's inside is not evident from the outside. Due to household changes starting tomorrow, tonight was my best window of opportunity for gift wrapping. However, Dale had therapy evaluations for several hours so I didn't feel I should make additional stops to try to find these odd boxes before getting him home. So, home we went, and within the first thirty minutes as we settled in, we had two separate packages delivered within ten minutes of each other... and, *yes, the packing boxes were exactly the two different sizes I needed!*

I have to smile. God knows me and knows my needs and the desires of my heart, even the smallest. And He knows when I need encouragement; it had been a hard morning. One of the deliveries was a bouquet of beautiful flowers! Thank you, Daddy, and thank you to those who listened and contributed to the perfect timing. The gifts are now wrapped, and we are blessed.

12/19/2015 Brain Changes

Our brain health friend visited for her first evaluation of Dale since the 12/3 stroke. Although I wanted her evaluation since it will give us a point of comparison, it is sad for me to watch and note the areas of regression. Lord, I come to You to release this sorrow and cast this care on You. Grieving - Lord, do You grieve as Your children move in distance from You? I think you would as You made humans in Your image and grieving is our natural, unjaded response.

12/20/2015 Birthday Musing

Good morning, Daddy. Thanks for the early birthday cup of tea, the beautiful star show and first light. You know that's my favorite time of day. I appreciate the reminder that You know when I sit and when I rise. You are familiar with all my ways. "He sees you when you're sleeping; He knows when you're awake" is not just describing Santa Claus! I trust You with my waking and with my rest.

12/25/2015 Christmas at Home

Last year at Christmas, Dale was at inpatient rehab in Tampa, and I was living in Brandon with his sister and brother-in-law and spending days at the rehab with Dale and four other brain-injured new friends. We made quite a "family" as we shared each other's lives and encouraged each step of progress. On Christmas Day 2014, Dale had his first overnight away from rehab at David's as we gathered our immediate family for precious time together under one roof, so thankful for a reprieve of only thirty-three hours.

So, after the recent stroke and ensuing weeklong hospital stay, we have cherished being HOME to heal, to recover and regroup, to settle and recharge, and to be loved. Since I had decorated for the holidays over Thanksgiving weekend, when we returned from the hospital December 10th, we readily soaked up the season's love, lights, and music, taking opportunities to look and listen, to sing and even dance a bit. We encourage you to do the same this Christmas Day; breathe deeply, look around and observe those around you, express your thankfulness (no matter if it can only be for the little things), give of yourself - your time, your attention, your love. None of us are guaranteed another day, even another moment, nor another opportunity to be with a loved one or to express love or appreciation.

Dale and I, along with our close family, had our lives changed in the timespan of a heartbeat at 10:00 p.m. October 3, 2014. *We were totally turned upside down.* I ask *"What will rock your world?"* Maybe something already has and you're reeling from it. In the midst of that life-storm, God knows; He's "got this." His plans for us do not end as we are hurt or suffer, as our mortal bodies decline nor as they pass away, rather His plans for us extend throughout the eternity we already inhabit. We've only just begun. You've likely heard, *"Yesterday is history. Tomorrow is a mystery. Today is a gift. That's why it's called the present."*

Take a moment today to reflect, to be a gift by being "present" with those around you, and make it a merry Christmas.

We love you and appreciate you. You are each precious to us both; we ask our Heavenly Father to bless you with wisdom, strength, peace, love and joy in abundance.

1/1/2016 Welcome 2016!

It's 3:50 a.m. and I've been awake for over an hour which is physically uncomfortable. I am hot, over-full, and have much on my mind. I sat on the porch (69 degrees) with my new flamingo throw and RESTED in God. Then, came in to reflect and record. I am now using my new chrome book light. It is perfect!

As health surrogate/helper, moving into 2016, I am to consider these in light of *new* post-stroke needs:
- order our days until Dale can contribute
- prayerfully consider what to do and delegate what I can
- check out LED/incandescent/halogen bulbs vs. fluorescent
- music/songs - RELAX playlist
- reorganize bedroom - essential oils, books, furniture

Reminders and insights:
- REST
- LAUGH
- SING
- <u>do not only sit</u> - MOVE, STAND
- be expansive, large in motion, exercise movements, dance, painting, swimming, BOSU

1/4/2016 Cracks and Brokenness

"There's a crack, a crack in everything that's how light gets in." - Leonard Cohen ('Anthem')

That reminded me of my great-niece's writing, *"Growth is not always easy, sometimes it means facing your brokenness and allowing the Lord to graciously take all your scattered pieces and form you into a beautifully broken vessel of his love, grace, and mercy. Only He can make this messy heart a joyful masterpiece."* May we welcome growth in every form over this next year.

Isaiah 28:12 "He is the Repairer of broken walls." He takes the broken (that He allows or even breaks as in the case of Jesus) and uses that broken person for His purposes. John 12:24 "Very truly I tell you, unless a kernel of wheat falls to the ground and dies, it remains only a single seed. But if it dies, it produces many seeds." In nature's process, seeds split open (break) to bring forth a new plant (new life). Once harvested, grain is crushed into flour to make bread which in turn gives sustenance (life) to others.

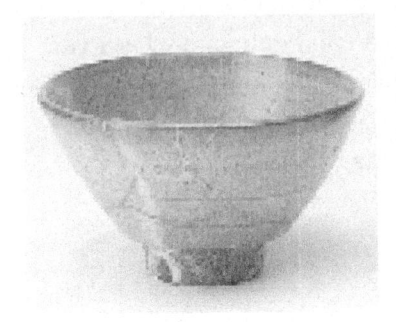

Kintsurkuroi provides a perfect example of this: the art of repairing pottery with gold or silver lacquer resulting in the repaired piece being more beautiful for having been broken.

Counting and recounting blessings:
- radiology tech from church who cared for/advised us
- Dale is home
- Steen family are here to help, bringing peace to our families
- computers are refreshed
- blue skies, clouds, and sunshine
- river view
- time to fast
- great team of doctors

Chapter Nine

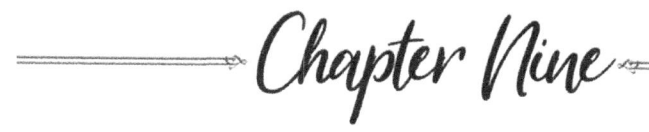

SHARED LIVES

1/16/2016 The Glorious Unknown

*The steps of a good man are **ordered by the Lord**, And He delights in his way.*   *Psalms 37:23*

So... Thursday, we experienced this once again. After spending the night in Sarasota for a sleep study (Dale has no sleep apnea diagnosis, praise God), we headed out for a full day only to have our appointments totally scrapped by 9:30 a.m.! Okay. Trusting God with our day, we moved forward visiting my sister Patti. During conversation, she told us of a "brain facility" she'd recently been made aware of right down the street from her and along the lines of what we'd all been reading about for several years. Interesting. I looked up their website and, noting that they took "walk-ins," called to see if they preferred walk-ins or appointments, only to find out that the founder and a nurse practitioner each had a free consultation slot available that afternoon, so I booked them! After meeting with the nurse practitioner, dietitian, and neurotherapist, and considering how to proceed, Dale is scheduled next week with the dietitian for thorough evaluation of diet intake, exercise schedule, and meds over three sessions, and with the doctor for a brain mapping followed by a series of ten neurofeedback sessions twice a week. In addition to an additional financial commitment (as these are not covered by insurance), it is also a big change in our weekly plans, driving to Sarasota two days for these appointments. We appreciate your prayers on our behalf for travel, outcomes, finances, and the relationships with these individuals.

Since the first of December, our life has been a continual series of ups and downs with many surprises of various sorts. I'm reminded of a story we heard years ago likening life with Jesus to a motorcycle ride where He invites us to hop on the bike behind him as He's driving—an unexpected, wild ride indeed.

I concur; life is definitely an adventure! Experiencing highs and low, the great unknown. Through it all, assurance of God's faithfulness. His surrounding of these times pervades my thoughts, my consciousness and likely my unconsciousness. We flow, changing and settling, changing and settling, again... again - good signs. *Life is growth*; it is said that growth is the only evidence of life.

To update you:

-After our first week at home in December, our dear longtime friends, Sam, Cyndi, and Hope Steen, moved in with us to help in any way possible with therapies, daily household upkeep, respite - anything that comes along.

-So... the second week home had all of us adjusting to living together. By Christmas Eve, however, I truly could feel the load lifted, and shifted, and the blessing of community living became a reality. All five of us have been there before, and it fits well.

-For the last two weeks of 2015, Dale had OT/PT/Speech twice a week at the same Englewood facility as last year—a good fit all around. Medicare took care of all these therapies, including Speech, through December 31st. Lots of progress, but no routine at all due to holidays. Sam worked with him for several hours each afternoon; bless him, Lord. It's an obvious benefit to have someone other than me coaching Dale and he's responding well, hallelujah.

-2016 promises new beginnings and we are grateful to see more of a pattern to our life over the first half of the month.

-Although Medicare will cover therapies in the near future, we know that will max out over the next few months so have organized this opportunity to Dale's advantage with OT and PT. Since speech is the main struggle and that we have already been working with an awesome therapist (and his team), we continue to put our financial resources into that endeavor; Dale resumed online sessions and we are thrilled. Sam is now Dale's main coach and is doing a superb job, adding his expertise and daily personal observation to the mix; Cyndi sits in on sessions as well and applies what she learns to our daily living. It's a very rich blessing to have four caring individuals conversing and interacting with Dale within the household instead of him only hearing my voice.

-Typically, Dale and I do a nutritional fast/cleanse twice a year, once usually in January after the holidays. This year's was spurred on both by a corporate fast called by our church and articles/Ted Talks on intermittent fasting and its benefits for the brain. So... we've embarked on eating only between the hours of 11 and 7, gone back to our clean eating lifestyle, and are fasting two low calorie days weekly for this month with our church. We enjoy feasting and comfort foods, but it is good to be back in the groove; Cyndi and Hope are spoiling us by cooking for the household - blessings on them.

-We've pretty much been singing/worshipping daily since we got home. That is one of the things the Lord impressed upon me as I sought His wisdom upon returning home:
   -fresh air and sunshine/out in nature
   -expansive exercise/large in motion
   -laugh
   -sing
   -do not only sit

These were our reminders. In addition to thanking and/blessing God, we now know that our singing and humming is wonderful for the brain, body, and nervous system.

Prayer needs:
- continued schedule changes as Dale moves forward and his therapies change
- our household interactions
- relationships with neighbors and medical team - those who need to know Father's love

2/26/2016 Since Some Have Asked...

Many times this month, it's been on my mind to connect with loved ones, yet priorities haven't allowed time to write in this journal. Consequently, we've had both friends and extended family ask for an update. Our entire household is well, thankfully, and in good health. Weather has been welcoming us to be outdoors, so we walk or exercise in the pool as we can in addition to workouts two to three times a week and are grateful for fresh air and sunshine and physically being able to exercise. We continue to follow our local grandsons' activities and enjoy the social interaction with many of their parents/grandparents that we've known for decades. These boys are a joy to watch, intent on playing well, coachable, polite, and good teammates; we are blessed to live nearby. We attend our church most weeks and listen to good audiobooks/teachings; we've watched many movies in the evenings along with recorded favorite TV shows, and we accept every social invitation that we can.

Dale progresses daily and for that we are most grateful. Little successes are acknowledged and applauded. They require much effort and energy for Dale's and those who are working with him.

Since I wrote last, Dale:

-has online speech therapy two times weekly and Sam is his primary coach the rest of the week. Dale requested to work with another therapist as well; next week he will begin alternating sessions with two SLPs. It's a great sign of progress to take personal responsibility and voice his preferences (leading his own therapy). In addition, Dale takes part in a group speech cafe once or twice weekly with a different therapist and a group of aphasics who are working on their speech in various ways; they've become friends.

-gave a presentation this past week to his speech cafe with the assistance of the therapist. We had produced a short PowerPoint of our 2011 Alaska trip. It was a great success.

-along with me, Dale completed our fast, had three visits with a nutritionist and have fine-tuned our eating, including more protein and more variety of foods. Visiting the local farmers' market is a favorite weekly outing. Driving to appointments in Sarasota several times a week has both caused us to plan meals accordingly and afforded us welcome opportunities to shop at Trader Joe's and Costco.

-has been to neurotherapist for initial brain mapping and subsequent twice-weekly neurofeedback sessions. We have seen continued clarity and speech progress throughout this time and are most grateful for this treatment and the doctor, who played rugby at UF while Dale was playing football and whose 101-yr-old father lives in Englewood and was able to attend a retired teachers' breakfast as our guest. God has given us many interesting connections!

-has primarily been coached by Sam in speech and visual/perceptual therapy; he has also been Dale's gym buddy during the time Dale was re-familiarizing himself with the equipment and routine. Sam's expertise and research abilities brought much-needed insights to both Dale and me that have greatly enhanced both the therapies and personal adjustments we've faced since the December stroke.

-rode with me to Naples to visit our daughter Christy and her new roommate, a dear family friend. It was a good time; we're thrilled they are living together and that they have cats! There was also time for Dale to have a "brain therapy" session and great improvement was noted.

Living with Dale 24/7, I especially have to remember that the stroke in December did new and additional damage to his brain, so some previous therapies have to be revisited, new neural pathways established, and some new areas now need therapy. He is not yet able to read in sentences as tracking is difficult, yet he can readily read individual words, even upside down as he sees them on cards. On the other hand, sometimes a familiar word or name is not retrievable without assistance; this changes with repetition and as new connections are formed, sometimes easily after one time through but other words take more repetitions. Word retrieval and all aspects of communication require much brain energy and are adversely affected as energy wanes.

Several times I've been asked, "What do you do with your days?" (a reference to being "retired"). This is laughable to those of you who've been in a caregiving position; others have no way of understanding. Even with the wonderful family support, and the assistance and company of the Steen family and all they undertake on our behalf, there is much to be done. So, my days are spent:
- encouraging, assisting, and supervising Dale
- reading informational books/articles/testimonials
- keeping up with scheduling and driving to doctor/therapy appointments – two to three times a week an hour away
- shopping for groceries and household needs
- assisting and guiding Dale in dressing and making choices
- in conversation about Dale's concerns and questions, all to help maintain his peace of mind

      -gauging Dale's energy level, encouraging rest time before overload and confusion set in

It's hard to explain how much time is needed to just to assist Dale and communicate with him. Thankfully, having the Steens here has given me the opportunity to leave the house as needed, providing respite for me and saving Dale from having to be traipsed all over town to run errands. I am most grateful for "retreat" times in my room or on the porch and for opportunities to walk, exercise and shop without the responsibility of supervising normal daily activities - simple things that mean so much.

Please continue to keep us in prayer:
      -we often face obvious spiritual battles with anxiety, fear, being "stuck" on a topic, impatience, and weariness. Galatians 6:9 "And let us not grow weary while doing good, for in due season we shall reap if we do not lose heart."
      -Dale has been taken off one medication (hallelujah!) and is in the middle of being weaned off sleep meds, causing adjustments and changes in body chemistry, a process that is likely to continue over the next few months.
      -a weekend family vacation is planned for March 11-13 and we ask for prayer as we travel by car and reacquaint ourselves with hotels and visiting new places. This short trip with family to support and enjoy is a trial run for future trips.
      -continued grace for our household living arrangements and discernment of each other's needs
      -relationships with neighbors and medical team; prayer for those who need to know Father's love

3/9/2016 Thorns and Roses

A thorny week, the hardest we've had since the December stroke, yet roses bloomed in the midst. My husband gave me beautiful flowers, definitely the prettiest assortment I've ever received. And our Good Neighbor Award goes to the couple who brought them to Dale so he could show how much he loves me. What a blessed act of kindness! It's heartwarming to be loved as you're engaged in battle. May God richly bless them as they blessed us.

4/4/2016 Another Month, Another Update

Spring is refreshing. It is my favorite time of year and we've been blessed with 'open windows' even this week; it's good for my soul.

After a full month of heavy therapy and two to four trips to Sarasota weekly (an hour drive), on April 1st we began a relaxed schedule, more at-home and rest-based. Dale has persevered in speech and neurofeedback all of February and March with OT as well until three weeks ago when OT was replaced by vision therapy. His progress has been evident on a daily basis and there are reconnections in many areas, too many to list; he is on the last leg of weaning off the night meds and has had checkups and good reports from his cardiologist, neurologist, and neurotherapist. We are SO grateful for these wonderful doctors, all of whom talk the medical talk with Dale face to face and encourage him to live life!

Physically, Dale is increasing his endurance and upping his cardio intensity (mildly intense at this point); He walks daily and goes to the Y for workouts twice a week. His self-monitoring has improved, acknowledging when he needs a rest and wisely doing so. Our daily therapy and household workload is greatly relieved by our dear friends and housemates; they are God's gift to our whole family.

Mentally and emotionally, both of us are challenged daily. We continue to learn about God's amazing design of the brain and implement new knowledge into the process of recovery. We've weathered many ups and downs this month, overall experiencing a lessening of anxiety. What a great blessing to all involved!

Relationally, we are healthy and united in our focus. Our household of five is thriving for however long God has us together under one roof. Conversation among many instead of just the two of us serves as the most obvious and natural means to encourage Dale's speech and ward off the specter of loneliness and discouragement.

Socially, we had a fabulous weekend with our kids and grandkids in St. Augustine at the beginning of Spring Break, visiting the old city and fort, watching a St. Patrick's Day parade complete with bagpipes and kilts, spending several hours together with one of my high school friends, and enjoying a fantastic evening meal at the Columbia Restaurant. That trip was a trial run for future travel, and we passed it with flying colors!

So, April 1st, we left for Dale's trip of choice, a sports weekend in Gainesville where we met up with our daughter Christy and grandson Joshua. In addition to enjoying Florida Relays (track) and Gator softball and tennis, we also were able to visit our dear family friends. As we travel, Dale and I are grateful we share so much history together; our road trips include music and audiobooks that we both enjoy. Gainesville is where we met, married, had our first home and first child, still a special town to us.

Spiritually, we depend on God's guidance, knowing we need it for every step. He is faithful to meet every need, pour out wisdom as we ask, and surround us with His comfort and love. It is a pleasure to have agreement in fellowship, worship, and prayer in our home.

5/26/2016 To Everything There is a Season...

In early April, we worked on balancing Dale's schedule, giving more space to heal through rest, relaxation, and recreation. In his present neural situation, everyday living situations are therapy in themselves; everything requires more effort and energy for him than for those of us who haven't had neurological damage. Just waking up in the morning immediately reminds him of his speech impairment, simply getting dressed challenges spatial and organizational brain functions, and any conversation provokes constant effort physically, mentally, and emotionally.

I've often used the analogy of a car transmission: those of us without TBI impairment function as an <u>automatic</u> transmission; Dale with the neural impairment from the stroke functions as a <u>manual</u> stick shift. Consider any new places, people, and crowded spaces with lots of movement and you get a sampling of how much energy he expends to simply navigate a new location.

So... we continue to evaluate the whole picture. This past week I ran across an old email from sixteen months ago when we were first returning home after four months of inpatient rehab. In it I stated:

> "<u>Dale's job</u> - to work hard at all aspects of rehab. <u>My job</u> - to be his wife/his help, to gather and assimilate rehab info and oversee the schedule, and to keep the household and financial aspects of our lives functioning peaceably."

Recognizing that I was inspired to address those goals as such, I'm grateful to look back and see the truth of those words. A constant part of my awareness is gauging Dale's energy level in hopes of encouraging rest time before overload and confusion set in. Thankfully, Dale's self-monitoring has been slowly increasing; there are times he recognizes his need for a "brain break." Both our "jobs" require a great expenditure of all of our personal resources—energy, wisdom, time, knowledge, and ability. I can feel just as impaired as Dale when I fall short in being able to help.

"And then there's GOD..." His resources are inexhaustible and His provision for us has been as overwhelming in its all-sufficiency as our personal energy and knowledge has been overwhelming in its insufficiency. At every turn, sometimes hourly, His care and provision for our needs has been available and evident. Our part, and right now mainly MY part, has been to tune in to which voice/Voice I'm hearing. The cares of this world clamor for our attention and express urgency; God's voice and direction patiently wait for me to listen and recognize the next step to take, one step at a time, never rushing or looking too far ahead. Often, at present, my responsibility is to speak Truth aloud to Dale during this time that his reasoning and cognition is still recovering.

This is where your prayers and encouragement are such an important part of our lives. My decades of relying on Dale's strengths to balance my own as we faced life's trials and made decisions together are now the foundation for what I face without his cognitive input to balance mine. Good counsel from my close family and friends, the prayers and resources from others, and God's welcome interjections through unexpected sources are now carrying us through as Dale continues in recovery. Our pastor prophesied four years ago when Dale retired from teaching and we prepared to return to Englewood that "we had given to so many for so long, and now it was our turn to receive." That was more than two years before Dale had a stroke, and it continues to unfold. Thank you for what you have given into our lives. It has definitely made me more mindful of specific and continued prayer for others.

Now for my personal exciting news; after eighteen months of constantly being on call with Dale, last week I was delighted and privileged to be able to take a three-night, four-day excursion to my hometown of Sackets Harbor, NY, with two of my sisters—the "Sackets' sisters"—Carol and Nancy, who share childhood memories of this wonderful but cold Snow Belt village. Can't say enough about our time in that precious lakeside town and the opportunity to reconnect with villagers there was both unexpected and heartwarming. *An excellent adventure!*

Those few days away not only provided me with much-needed R&R but also with an opportunity for fresh and new perspectives and observations as I returned. Upon reentry back into daily life, I had much to ponder. Thankfully, Dale did wonderfully well on "vacation" at home with the Steens, although THEY appeared to be in need of respite upon my return. So be it... God had already arranged for them to have this Memorial Day weekend with a friend as we are in Orlando with our grandsons.

Our goals are to learn more, live life, and make a difference for others. Sometimes it's recognizing a need in others; other times it's simply pushing to take another step instead of giving up. All the while, we remain grateful even in those moments we feel helpless, continuing to look up, and giving thanks to God for:
-family and friends
-laughter
-fresh air, sunshine, and a river view
-lighter traffic in the summer
-increasing knowledge on the brain
-an awesome team of therapists/helpers
-flashes of inspiration that stop us in our tracks
-and for lilacs! ...having just come from NY

7/2/2016 Blessings in the Midst...

Seems like a regular pace is most needed for the summer, still acknowledging our norm to remain flexible. Dale is working with a personal trainer for the next few months to build organization into his workouts, gain more muscle tone, and improve endurance. With his brain's executive function still recovering, this seems to be a timely answer. The facility is in the same building as vision therapy, so we are in Sarasota two days a week and also schedule in time for massage with sister-in-law Melodie, twice-a-month aphasia support reading group, running errands, or visiting family. That's our summer routine with two days of speech and home therapy, a break day on Wednesdays and weekends, and time with Christy, David's family, and local friends. We have no travel plans till mid-August. There have been many changes over the past month with both ups and downs. Dale is finally totally weaned off sleep meds, a five-month process, and we are grateful; he is sleeping well. This has freed his brain to recognize his present situation more clearly, which also brings both emotion and frustration with how long recovery can take. He's also admitted being scared and all of the household has helped him to overcome during those hard times.

God is faithful to show us the next step. I truly only need His answer for this moment's need and continue to learn to listen just for *that*, not jumping ahead in my wondering. His answer for each moment's needs is often JUST FOR THAT MOMENT whereas our nature is to want to look ahead. He promises DAILY bread and reminds us to NOT WORRY about tomorrow (I love the Old Testament example of just enough manna for a day!). *That's my focus.*

It's been a tough week and I'm evaluating many things along with Sam, looking at things circumspectly and slowing down when we don't know what to do. Our household/family are involved in a spiritual battle and it's evident. Sam and Cyndi have been counseling a couple—very fruitful and timely—and we've all been aware of battling many things. Victories on several fronts in the household and with others, too, so we're aware of the enemy's devices and are given more to prayer and praise. A mutual friend had a mild small stroke recently and his navigation skills have been affected; I hope to be able to help his wife in learning more, even about what to ask. And a lady in our condo village lives with her adult son who was impaired with something from his childhood; he had a stroke

Wednesday and is hospitalized; we're in touch and waiting to see how we can be of help and encouragement. Friendships with other stroke survivors and their spouses are strengthening and that has brought a measure of fulfillment and purpose.

In the midst of our trials, blessings! Today we were financially blessed to get a cottage king room with a lanai at Boca Grande's Gasparilla Inn for our 45th anniversary next weekend; we are excited! We'll go down Friday afternoon and leave Sunday, probably in time for church. Then we'll attend a retirement party for a teacher friend that afternoon. It will be a nice weekend, no matter the weather! We are blessed; thank you, God.

I love living in Englewood where we have rich history and are connected with so many wonderful people! Glad for blessings and the encouragement they bring, for God's faithfulness, for summer vacations for our kids, and for good sleep... and for the Steens being here to love us, share the load, pray, and offer some relief.

Hope your summer is wonderful and that you enjoy celebrating the 4th, remembering those who fought for our freedom and continue to serve to that end.

8/9/2016 Summer Progress...and Prayer Needs

We have finished two months of summer schedule and Dale has progressed (with the assistance of his physical trainer) in endurance and muscle tone from his twice-weekly workouts. In addition, he is noticeably more active in his pool. He is walking and plays a good game of ping-pong nearly every day. Speech continues to become more fluent; yet, pronunciation is best with fewer words, so communication continues to be a challenge, especially when Dale is tired or emotional. Vision therapy has helped him track in reading, and perception continues to improve slowly as does cognition and

A Caregiver's Journal

spatial location. We continue to work on his sense of order and time/hours/days; numbers and money have still not been restored at this point.

> **NOTE:** As the person who actually got to play that daily ping-pong game - for months - with Dale, Sam noted that in addition to enjoying daily morning walks filled with genuine, flowing conversations (complete with identifications and imitations of local wildlife) as well as golden oldie songs and nonstop charades, we do well to highlight Dale's extraordinary level of motivation and energy he brought to those times of "therapeutic fun" as *they* called it. That late spring through early summer was Dale's best, even happiest, season of self-improvement, a time when he was often feeling really great about himself and his progress, and justifiably so. It did him a world of good, and it filled him with encouragement to see the fruit of his labors come through in natural interactions. And we were simply 'living life' by walking, playing, communicating, recreating, and having fun doing it. Emphasizing that is very important, because it could have been quite easy, with all the changes and losses that Dale went through, to get mired in the downer aspect of things. But we incorporated making progress into all of the fun and games and interpersonal time. Through all of it, Dale was very much *just being himself*. And he enjoyed that feeling; that and seeing the hard work paying off. So, ping-pong was *also* our time for working on improving Dale's visuospatial perception, skills and movement integration. Relaxed walking-and-talking was *also* a great time for overcoming apraxia, while pursuing a broad range of topics that were of personal interest to Dale. Far from being a chore, it was a pleasure. And that was entirely attributable to Dale's positive, "can do"

attitude during those fun times. **It's vital for people to know that they can experience the same sort of manifold benefit.**"

The Suncoast Aphasia Support Group out of Sarasota has provided a bright spot in our social interactions and also hosts a reading group that we attend twice a month. Most of you reading this probably don't realize how our social life has changed, even with caring family and friends. Aphasia presents a tremendous strain on relationships and is exhausting for even the closest family members. Consequently, visits are fewer, phone calls can hardly happen, and our social time is most comfortable with those who have had similar experiences. It's a strange occurrence that takes its toll on relationships over time; we are thankful for those who are supportive and prayerful and count it a great a blessing to have relationships, both new and old, that bear with Dale's special needs. So, family gatherings, church, and support group functions are especially dear to us and we both look forward to each event. Dale's favorite activity is still to watch sporting events, especially those in which our grandchildren are involved or Christy's volleyball team.

We have also learned much about emergency services and what is required for Dale to contact 9-1-1 when he doesn't use a phone, type or write, and cannot be understood clearly when he speaks. Imagine that for a moment and realize that whenever he's alone with me or any one person, the reality exists that he might need emergency assistance should something happen to the one he's with. As I asked others in similar situations what their emergency plan was, it truly shocked me to find they really didn't have a realistic emergency plan in place! So, as I set out to learn what would meet our personal needs, I was asked to check out resources for the benefit of others. God had graciously gone before me and connected me with wonderful and caring individuals who helped put the pieces of this puzzle together, and I immediately felt a sense of purpose to help others with these special needs. So, we move forward, step by step, grateful for what we do have and for the many things we CAN do.

The Steen family is still living with us and I cannot tell you what a blessing it is to have others to daily share life with us. God only knows how long they'll be here. I don't fear life with just the two of us, but as we look toward the possibility of buying a home, a supportive community is at the very top of our list of needed assets. Until you live "in our shoes," it is hard to grasp what our life is like (and it's exhausting to describe or explain).

Prayer request: It is 3:00 a.m. as I write this and we leave mid-morning to fly to Columbus, OH, for a two-week visit with Nancy and Ken. Travel, change, and new surroundings all present new challenges for us and, consequently, new opportunities for growth and brain reconnections. Please keep us and them in your prayers as we cross your mind. We do look forward to time together, for a "vacation break" from routine, from therapy, and even from home surroundings, time to relax and reflect. We expect God's refreshing and direction. He is SO faithful to lead me/us in even the small things: this morning I was reminded to leave the house early enough to get new wiper blades put on. After doing so, within thirty minutes, I drove through the greatest blinding downpour so far this year!

God is our Refuge and God is our Strength, a very present help in trouble. He MAKES me lie down in green pastures; He LEADS me beside still waters; He restores my soul. I praise and thank Him for His great love and for Who He is and that He knows everything that concerns me. I trust Him. Furthermore, I truly thank God upon every remembrance of you and consider it a privilege to pray for you and yours, even in the wee hours of the night.

August Notes, 2016

Vacation at Nancy and Ken's was a blessed time of relaxing and refreshing—outstanding home and hospitality, neighborhood, and landscape. Dale has been weaned off Seroquel completely since May except for a small dose when traveling. I am grateful to report that this vacation was good for us both and no anxiety surfaced.

We had a smooth and successful flight to Columbus, and a week later (8/23/2016), a good flight home - our first flights since Dale's second stroke event. Interestingly, "post-stroke Dale" accepted ATL wheelchair assistance without questions or irritation; uniforms on escorts were an asset. However, Dale's ears were really painful on the flight back from changes in cabin pressure. Not good.

> **IMPORTANT NOTE YEARS LATER: In retrospect, I would be VERY cautious about flying. Although the planning and actual logistics of navigating new spaces together can be successful, our experiences have shown that the effects of altitude and pressurized air in the cabins have likely been sources of problems in Dale's brain that caused additional (and unnecessary) trauma provoking anxiety and resulting in extremely distraught behavior. Sadly, only in hindsight was I able to discern this, and not even after this first flight. These next entries detail what I now consider (years later) to be at least partially due to the effects of air travel. I pray that others learn from our experiences.**

8/24 - Dale awoke in the morning startled and talking about dogs... none around.

8/25 - after retiring at 11:00 p.m., he was awake at 2:00 a.m. for about an hour. He was distraught about pills and water, "dead," and said hateful things to me. This woke Hope up in the other room, so I told her to get her parents up. At some point, Dale started talking to Sam, but before that I called David because Dale was so hateful, and he listens well to David. But he didn't even believe David although David reinforced truth. Finally after an hour, Dale was exhausted, and Sam was able to help him settle. He slept another hour, then used the bathroom normally and slept again so I closed our door, but I didn't sleep much – about four hours. We went to Sam's Club after breakfast, but he tired quickly and slept for over an hour when we got home at 10:30 a.m. His behavior was normal but he was tired, watched a movie with Sam, and we went to Naples for a volleyball game. He enjoyed singing oldies in the car and the volleyball game then had a good ride home. He watched the Tonight Show and went to bed at 11:00 p.m.

8/26 – Dale awoke at 3:00 a.m. to use the bathroom (normal); woke again at 4:00 a.m. distraught and asked for Sam. Dale had same confused, strange, and fixated behavior. He then slept until nearly 10:00 a.m. but then awoke distraught and accusing for over an hour. It was a very hard day. We watched a music special and attended a memorial service for a young man, a former student/football player of Dale's; we saw many people who are special to Dale/us. By the time we got home, he was distraught again, not surprising for many reasons. Thankfully, we had a peaceful evening.

8/27 - SO glad praise is part of the testimony as we walk with God. Dale had a wonderful night's sleep and I revisited the possible need for "night pills" if/as needed. I am thankful for freedom in the Lord to be flexible, not rigid or feeling condemnation for my actions or decisions. THIS IS HARD. There was no stress this morning, but Dale is still needing sleep and is napping on the couch again at 11:30 a.m. after normal exercise/activity. Praise God. We had a normal day and went to sleep readily at 10:00 p.m. after the Rays' game. He was very discerning and asked for audio Scriptures!

8/28 -Dale slept normally until 5:00 p.m., then awoke distraught for nearly an hour, although settled faster. He was threatening to me, although I had given him a "night pill" early on for the first time. I was not afraid, but aware and conscious to speak Truth and not allow lies to linger in the air. Also, I was mindful to bring everything to light with no shame and give the enemy NO place, so I shared incident details with the Steens and later with my kids. Overall, it was a good day as we had David's birthday dinner and caught up with happenings. It is always a pleasure and respite for me and the household to have family visit as they so readily take responsibility for Dale/Papa in conversation and activity and the household gets a mental break as well as enjoying our family interaction. Dale went to bed early and sought out Sam for conversation before retiring.

8/29 – We had full normal night's sleep. Hallelujah!

> **NOTE: Not long after this, Dale was set free from fear. However, we choose to acknowledge it—physically, spiritually, mentally, emotionally—in looking back, it seems evident that air travel played a part and, in my opinion, should be approached with great caution.**

9/3/2016 Guidance

It is SO evident that without You Lord, I can do nothing. I have NO idea how to relate to Dale and yet we are still one and I still know him better than anyone else. Yet, I can't understand him, can't truly put myself in his place although I try; he can't explain needs and feelings; I can't seem to help him; he's so unhappy and it has become a continual battle for me to fight the negativity that comes from him.

Wisdom/encouragement from Romans 8:18, esp. 26-28,35-39 and then Romans 12:1-5 and:

v. 6-8 Having then gifts differing <u>according to the grace that is given to us...let us use it in our ministering</u>;
- he who exhorts, in exhortation;
- he who gives, with liberality;
- he who leads, <u>with diligence</u>;
- he who shows mercy, <u>with cheerfulness</u>.
- Abhor what is evil. Cling to what is good.

v. 10 - Be kindly affectionate to one another with brotherly love,
- in honor giving preference to one another;

v. 11 - not lagging in diligence,
- fervent in spirit, <u>serving the Lord</u>

v. 12 - <u>rejoicing</u> in hope,
- <u>patient</u> in tribulation,
- <u>continuing steadfastly in prayer</u>;

v. 13 - distributing to the needs of the saints,
- (be) given to hospitality.

v. 14 - <u>Bless</u> those who persecute you; bless and do not curse.

v. 15 - Rejoice with those who rejoice; with those who weep.

v. 16 - associate with the humble. Don't be wise in your own eyes.

v. 17 - Repay no one evil for evil.

v. 18 - If it is possible, <u>as much as depends on you</u>, live peaceably with all men.

v. 19 - do not avenge yourselves...

v. 20 - "If your enemy is hungry, feed him; If he is thirsty, give him a drink..."

v. 21 - Do not be overcome by evil, but overcome evil <u>with good</u>.

Chapter Ten

TWO YEARS OF CHANGED LIVES

10/3/2016 It's Been Two Years

Two years ago today, Dale and I were traveling to Hilton Head for a getaway with my sister and brother-in-law. I had just retired from my twenty-six-year job as a yearbook rep three days earlier and we were getting out of town! That night at 10:00 p.m. during our stay over in Amelia Island, our lives were totally turned upside down when Dale suffered a massive ischemic stroke and had to be airlifted to UF Shands Jacksonville, not to return home again for four months. Ten months ago, on December 2, 2015, he suffered another, milder stroke; this time medical personnel were able to find Atrial Fibrillation as the source of the blood clots and to prescribe medication to dissolve any possible future clots. Hallelujah!

I know we've both been blessed over these two years by the love and support of our family and friends, by connections and relationships with wonderful therapists and medical personnel, and by the rich history we've shared in our forty-five plus years together. This shared history has proven to be especially meaningful as Dale has become more prolific in his thoughts and social interactions, often recounting anecdotes, or appropriate knowledge he wants to share regarding the situation at hand. **We are changed.**

Although Dale has always had a great sense of humor, he now more freely expresses his emotions through infectious laughter, even silliness. Children and animals stop him in his tracks as he gives them his full attention and revels in their antics, and he more freely sheds tears, often moved by touching personal stories from others' lives. My understanding simply put, is that since his brain damage was in the left hemisphere, the right hemisphere activity compensated, giving freer expression to his emotions and creativity.

As for me, I've learned more than I ever expected to or wanted about insurance, patient advocacy, medical protocols, hardships the medical profession faces, living with brain injuries, and the needs of co-survivors/caregivers. I've also learned to more deeply depend on God, for EVERYTHING. He is my Source: security, provision, wisdom, direction, peace, joy, and hope. I've grown in patience, perseverance, boldness, courage, in waiting and in hearing the voice of God. Since early in our marriage, Dale has described me as being content wherever I am; even more so over these two years. I have been tried through many living situations. I am at home where God has me; He is Home. It's the inward, not the outward, that I need to examine continually, and which causes me to trust Him and to change my heart as needed. He has already given us His peace; I simply need to allow myself to receive it.

"Search me, O God, and know my heart; test me and know my anxious thoughts. See if there is any offensive way in me, and lead me in the way everlasting." Psalm 139:23-24

We continue to move forward. Dale's speech is much more fluent, many words/phrases are understandable. His SLP continues to amaze us with his on-target suggestions; we so appreciate his depth of experience. And of course, Dale's total communication continues to improve as he relaxes and readily incorporates gestures and body language. Physically, his summer sessions with a personal trainer were successful in regaining muscle tone and increasing endurance. For that we are grateful and he'll continue workouts twice a week. October marks the beginning of new therapy goals, particularly in vision. Having been to a neuro-ophthalmologist, it's been confirmed that Dale's eyes and vision are good and in no further need of correction; the doctor encouraged Dale to remain in vision therapy for continued restoration of perception and cognitive issues. He also reminded us that *the recovery "clock" is reset from the last stroke*; in Dale's case, that is now ten months.

> *I am at home where God has me; He is home. He has already given us His peace; I simply need to allow myself to receive it.*

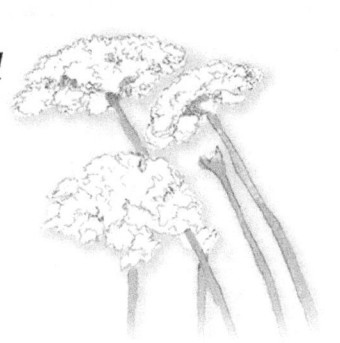

We ask for your prayers as we prepare for upcoming adjustments. Our friends the Steens are formulating their next move; they've been living with us since last December, coaching Dale and handling the household, so it will be a big shift to it being just the two of us again. Dale and I are also in the process of moving closer to town and purchasing a home in a retirement community with nearby neighbors and activities within walking distance.

Our family and friends are wonderful and so important to us. Your visits, notes, calls, and little surprises encourage and revive our spirits. As we are able, we visit, contact and pray for others, hoping to give love and encouragement. It is a joy to give back to others. Know you are loved and let us hear from you as time permits.

11/7/2016 Another Outburst...

On 11/5, after a full and enjoyable day (except for the Gator FB loss), we were unwinding with the TV. We had visited Boca Grande (where Dale tired from walking, but with no real breakfast), the drive home, lunch, then football. So, instead of directing him to rest fully and take a brain break, I let him watch from the couch, hoping he'd fall asleep. THAT DID NOT HAPPEN. Sam suggested ping-pong, then we caught about ten minutes of shuteye before going to David's. Dale was exhausted by the end of the game, and it was showing. He was then a bit restless while winding down at home.

A marked change occurred when he brushed his teeth and came out of the bathroom. I can now describe it as overload—a circuit shorted or like flipping a switch and the power going out. The next six hours were horrific as he "lost it."

- didn't know his home
- walked into the parking lot in the dark and yelled for help
- hit Sam
- was hateful in most of what he did to me/us
- rambled on in speech
- searched the house for familiar and to orient himself
- "shot" at us and things with his "finger gun"
- spoke death in several forms
- refused to go to bed

This was the night of the time change—fall back—so I stayed up with him until midnight. As I began to recognize that overstimulation and lack of sleep was in play, I gave him .625mg – ¼ of a 25mg. tablet of Seroquel that took about an hour to settle.

> **NOTE: Oh, how I wish I recognized these things sooner—the long days and that he's not self-evaluating as well as he had been. I would have adjusted our days offering fewer activities with longer breaks in between. I've had to grieve that and not blame myself for what I did not know. THIS is why I am freely sharing the hard times - the ugly and the hateful, so that others might gain**

from our experiences and apply knowledge sooner to their own situations.

He finally went to sleep at midnight, awoke at 3:00 a.m. and was still agitated, restless, and hateful for 1¼ hours. I was reminded of the Lord's word for me to sing praises aloud when Dale is upset, so I did in the midst of following him to the living room since it was dark and unsafe for him, back and forth from there to the bedroom. He ended up lying down with the lights on. Not long after, I was singing "Where Can I Go From Your Spirit" and began weeping. Dale reached over to comfort me; I could tell he was settled so when he asked me to lie down, I did, asking him if I could turn the lights off and Scriptures on. He agreed and slept well until 8:30 a.m.

He was only a little disoriented during the next day. We went to church where many encouraged us and prayed, then got lunch and drove to a favorite park to talk and walk. Later, we had a surprising and wonderful visit with dear friends who just stopped by.

12/6/2016 What Can I Do?

Oh, God, help me to hear You and not do things/step out on my own. This all-encompassing caregiving for Dale is so tenuous, so fragile in temperament, and in emotional ups and downs. I don't know why I assume I know what to do or what he needs or what is best. I truly know so little and yet want to do so much.

Thank you, Lord, for reminding me that You live right inside Dale and Your angels always are on assignment with him. He has Your provision. "It is not good for man to be alone"; that is my role; to be with him in this time. It became evident today through Dale's actions and discussion with Sam that I need to be discerning of the specific help I can offer Dale (we all need that discernment). Please pray for:

-Dale's discernment; it's developing to grasp what help he needs and doesn't need. That is progress; yet, self-evaluation wanes when he's tired and that is sometimes a quick shift
-wisdom for our household/family to know the difference
-us all to trust You to do Your part and show each of us ours

12/11/2016 Learning...

Well, I'm learning... a little more each day...
Last night, Dale had an anxiety episode that revealed to us the deep trauma from old events that surface when confronted with flashing lights such as fire trucks, police cars, ambulances, and tow trucks. As I recounted the scene, a tow truck with flashing lights came into the condo parking lot while Dale was out walking at dusk. We both immediately realized the connection between those flashing lights and Dale's ensuing anxiety as he spoke about being hit and being scared. There is no way to prepare for "emergency" vehicles showing up but we will talk about them as the occasions happen.

12/14/2016 "50 First Dates"

Steens had suggested the movie *50 First Dates*, and watching it provided lots of food for thought. Aside from the crude language typical of an Adam Sandler comedy, the story hit very close to home. I found myself thinking about it all the next day - an odd source of information and education for me.
    -TBI survivor perspective
    -caring family and friends
    -overprotectiveness vs. growth/change
    -inspired ideas (using videos of occasions)
    -repetition as a means to gain understanding and move forward more quickly
    -patience and love of family and friends overshadows all

Chapter Eleven

A NEW HOME

4/21/2017 The Past Six Months

Well, this turned out to be a long entry! It's been six months since my last entry and MUCH has happened in the past six months! Life was a whirlwind for a few months while we prepared to move to a new house. We've now been in this home two months, since February, and are relatively settled.

The move: Moving was Dale's request and he desired to be closer to the old Englewood area. *In reality, the actual process of uprooting and relocating is a major stressor for anyone, doubly hard for a caregiver, and overwhelming for any person with TBI issues.*

> **NOTE:** Moving is an ENORMOUS undertaking. Looking back, I've seen many advantages and disadvantages in our move, some of which you'll realize as you read through this part of the journal. As any caregiver considers a move, especially with a care-needing person who has communication or memory issues, it will be VITAL to enlist the candid counsel of your support circle. Moving home locations is hard work in anyone's life - physically, mentally, emotionally, socially; it is exponentially difficult with one who can give no assistance, still needs 24/7 care, and has no way of gauging how the move in total will affect him/her personally. All of that has to be assessed and carefully

weighed by the caregiver, family, and support circle. Once the decision is made to move locations, circumspect thinking and planning are of the utmost importance for every facet of the transition.

<u>In the case of our decision to move, the following factors strongly came into play:</u>
- Dale's unprovoked request to move "back to town"
- my lifelong practice of acknowledging God's hand in directing Dale for our family's provision and protection as we made important decisions together prayerfully. At this point, Dale's difficulty in communicating made his requests that much more important to consider seriously; his struggle to make them known signified their importance to him.
- at this point we had 24/7 trustworthy live-in assistance from the Steens for care, therapy, and household upkeep as well as help for packing and preparing the new house
- financially this was feasible including hiring movers
- our family and support circle were in agreement

<u>Factors that were beyond anyone's control were:</u>
-Dale's understanding/lack of it in the moving process
-his confusion being immersed in the unfamiliar new house, having no reference point and having no home base or centering place in his mind

In hindsight, the only thing I would have done differently would have been a slower weaning from the family who lived with us after the physical move to the new house. I now believe it would have been in Dale's best interests to have more people around on a daily basis as he was accustomed, even if it was only daytime. That could have served to help his transition to house, and then fewer people, rather than both at once.

Several years later, and after Dale had passed, I came to realize that Dale's motivation for this move very likely included his preparation and provision for me to live my future single life in a safe community environment in the heart of our hometown. **That "big picture" thoroughness was at the very core of Dale Hutcherson, family man, and for that I am continually thankful.**

> *The actual process of uprooting and relocating is a major stressor for anyone, doubly hard for a caregiver, and overwhelming for any person with TBI issues.*

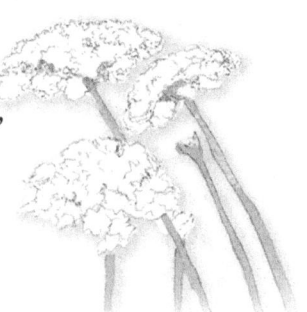

Although I had wonderful and continual assistance in preparing the house and caring for Dale... and we left town while the movers did the heavy work, the fact remains that such an upheaval takes its toll. When we got to the new house and Dale asked for things, I quickly realized within two days that <u>for Dale's stability, **everything** needed to be **out of boxes**</u> where I could at least locate it by sight, even if it didn't yet have a permanent place to "live." **For Dale, the move was like turning his brain map on end; everything he owned was in a new place, very little was familiar, and with his vision issues, new and multiple doors and openings were a constant source of confusion.** For the first three weeks, he didn't want to be there and asked to go "home," but not to the former condo. *"Home" meant familiar, normal... and he was struggling without it.* Routine gave some comfort and we maintained personal activities, speech therapy, and workouts purposefully, but also wanted him to have time to explore and settle. There was much to work through, many tears for us both. And the Steen family did not move with us to this new home, so navigating such great change with interaction just between the two of us was a HUGE and exhausting endeavor.

After settling in: Dale's great pleasure was watching our grandsons' sports, so we spent many afternoons watching tennis practice. Evenings continued to be for winding down, and during that time, we determined to watch comedies, knowing we both needed some time to be lighthearted. God was faithful in providing enough timely help from so very many sources and we were thankful for regular visits with our kids and grandkids.

During the fourth week home, Dale asked to talk with his sister Kim and said he was ready for a visit, so they came for the day and we began having visitors as part of our normal life once again. Anxiety lessened and tearful times were fewer in number, praise God. Nearly every day we are out and about for one reason or another, not at all housebound and thankful for that. We belong to two support groups and gain so much from the life experiences of others. We continue to walk through any door open to us, trusting God to open and close them. Many wonderful people have crossed our paths, some brief and blessed encounters; others developing into fruitful relationships. It is still our pleasure to help others, especially families and students, and we will freely share our story as opportunities arise.

Early this month we were guest speakers for the third time for FGCU's occupational therapy program, talking with students for two hours about what to expect when working with stroke survivors and their families and how they can help. The students are wonderful, many have personal experience with family or friends who need caregivers, and they ask great questions.

News and updates:

-The 2016 holidays were a pleasure, basically since we had been in rehab during the past two Decembers. So even in our crowded condo, we enjoyed celebrating with family and friends, went to Orlando for Thanksgiving, and gathered at David's for Christmas.

-Our friends the Steens lived with us for nearly fourteen months, helping in every possible way with therapy and household, providing five-way and often lively conversation, friendship, and respite. Once we moved into the new house, they continued with their own life.

-Speech therapy continues to be a focus. Dale is still having online sessions weekly with SLPs along with several online cafes and the Suncoast Aphasia reading group twice a month. We just finished a semester of free classes for aphasics at USF in Tampa and have **high praise for that program**. Dale loved it and I had a Caregivers' class as well. Definitely worth the weekly trip! In June, Dale is scheduled to participate in an Intensive Speech program at USF Tampa three hours a day Monday, Wednesday, and Friday for four weeks. We're looking forward to changing things up a bit for that month, taking a break from other speech therapies.

-Vision therapy continues, interrupted for a break doing only home exercises during the move. A trip to the neurologist-ophthalmologist in March showed Dale to have improved enough in hand-eye connections during the past six months to get an accurate field of vision test which showed obvious deficits on the left side of both eyes—left homonymous hemianopsia. Dale's reading ability is intact; he can read words fine, but has poor scanning left and right, consequently little motivation to read. We are beginning to work with Lighthouse for the Blind so he can get assistance in learning how to compensate for the deficits. A bonus is that he will now be getting Talking Books and the accompanying reading device, giving him another measure of independence.

New venture for prayer: I just finished reading *The Ghost in My Brain* for the second time and feel like it's timely to pursue brain and vision therapy with the two cutting-edge doctors highlighted in the book: Dr. Donalee Markus, a cognitive restructuring specialist (see Appendix One), and a colleague Dr. Deborah Zelinsky, an optometrist emphasizing neural optometric rehabilitation (see Appendix One). They are both located in Chicago about fifteen minutes from each other and I've made contact with both offices already. We will have to go for a five-day period, need someone to travel with us, and need the finances to make this happen. Will update on this Chicago trip when we know more.

Exercise is important; Dale walks daily and has weight training twice a week with a personal trainer who actually serves more as a workout buddy to keep Dale on the routine, to count reps aloud, and maintain safety with weight amounts and equal balance on both sides (Dale still has cognitive/perceptual issues). A blessing since Christmas break is that our oldest grandson Joshua has been Dale's workout partner as his schedule permits; he makes a little money on this, and we save a little; Papa is thrilled! Just yesterday a friend purposely told us how much improvement she'd seen in Dale at the gym; it's SO good to have an outside perspective! And, we just purchased a recumbent trike and Dale is thrilled to be motoring "alone;" he leads and I follow. Expecting great things as he builds endurance and confidence in navigation.

Dale successfully continues with guitar sessions weekly. His goal is to play Amazing Grace for his friends and family by himself.

We continue to read up on health/brain research and encourage everyone to read "Brain Maker" by Dr. David Perlmutter which documents the brain/gut connection. He is from Naples where we lived for ten years, and we know several who went to him and/or knew him. He is a practical neurologist who keeps up with whole body health research to implement in his patients' recovery.

In late December, we met Dr. Bo Martinsen of Omega 3 Innovations https://omega3innovations.com. We had been using his top-quality fish oil for about a year (incorporated it into our health regimen as soon as we learned about it. It is the best we've found!) and were told of the new developments in reintroducing melatonin back into the fish oil. Dale immediately started on it and results have been obvious in several areas—sleep, energy, calmer demeanor, and fine motor skill improvement. In the midst of all this we went to three excellent concerts:

Scan here for more information

  -Blood, Sweat, and Tears actually came to our little town and we sat in the second row. They were outstanding; Bo Bice (American Idol runner-up to Carrie Underwood) is a perfect new front man for them, doing justice to David Clayton Thomas songs and adding a few of his own.

  -Ethan Bortnick, a fourteen-year-old piano prodigy wowed our whole family with his talent and stage presence.

  -tobyMac, one of our favorites since we first heard of DCTalk in the late 80s, put on a blockbuster show with seven other artists/groups. We went with the whole family and friends and were up way past our bedtime... loved it!

Chapter Twelve

HARD TIMES

4/25/2017 My Update to Doctors

NOTE: since last October, there have been subtle changes in Dale's emotions/anxiety and his personal self-evaluation. Marking another year, some decline is noted by those close to him. Vascular dementia appears to be progressing and affecting these changes as well as Dale's ability to recognize safe/unsafe situations.

My update to his doctors - *I hand this note to the staff as we arrive for his appointment:*

In early February, we moved to a new home. The adjustment was very hard for Dale, like turning his brain map on end. He didn't know where to find any of his belongings or rooms in the house. He was confused and didn't want to be here, asking to go "home," but not the former condo, just wanting familiar, normal. It was heartbreaking. After three weeks, he was settled, still not finding rooms or things easily, but peaceful. **He definitely had setbacks in speech and cognition during that time, possibly in vision as well.**

Then, **two months out, early in April, Dale began having occasional episodes of anger and hatefulness, especially toward me, accompanied by restlessness and "tearing up" the room. He's left the house twice (and got out of the car once), wandering about the neighborhood.** I know he can't find his way home, so I follow after him from a distance until he's tired enough to be more compliant. After he "comes out of it," he is pleasant and more relaxed. There have been some bathroom issues, too like asking for help to how to sit on toilet and to find the toilet paper. Also, there have been some minor changes in eating. He can't seem to understand a sandwich or wrap, but takes items out of it.

> **NOTE: These are tough for me to see but Dale is seemingly not bothered by any of this or aware of these changing needs. A major change in our outings is that I need to identify public restrooms where I can be with him to assist him as needed. Newer facilities often have "family" restrooms or a single handicapped restroom, but many, even including malls and restaurants have NONE in individual stores or main bathrooms. Those of you with wheelchair use are likely already aware of this, but I hadn't faced it until now.**

My kids recognize these changes but basically I'm the one with him alone most of the time, although we do many things out of the house. **We'd like to have another brain MRI to see what might have changed since December 2015 or if there's anything additional that we're dealing with; however, it is likely we will simply (or not so simply) have to adjust to the decline. So sad.** Our family is not easily given to him being hospitalized for tests, etc., because that would be traumatic for him with aphasia and vision issues plus he has some residual fears from the first stroke experience. Additionally, I would need to stay at the hospital with him as well.

Neuro-ophthalmologist appointment last month successfully administered field of vision test (which Dale was not able to take accurately six months ago) and it showed **deficits on the left side of each eyeball—left homonymous hemianopsia**. Dale has been in vision therapy since last May, but it is slow moving, and we just resumed it this month after Dale was settled from our move. He likes this therapy, and the therapist is excellent; however, as I watch what he can and can't accomplish, the functional deficits Dale now has are very obvious and that is <u>very</u> emotional for me.

Also have noticed a few lethargic times and called cardiologist to learn more about AFib and what symptoms look like. **Dale's self-awareness is highly impaired and without him being able to evaluate how he feels, I'm left with only my observations, and that often delays the recognition.** I need to know the practical side of how to live with AFib and **would appreciate your advice.**

Dale no longer easily grasps medical conversation as he quickly latches onto either what he does understand and loses attention, or fears that change might mean another stroke or death. So, *I request that any discussion of change or medication be addressed with me alone and thank you for working with me on that since Dale is only frustrated by those decisions.* **Family is involved in all medical decisions; we talk with Dale at home when he's relaxed.**

Thankfully, Dale's doctors and their staffs were very understanding and helpful with this.

> **NOTE: MY OWN TRAUMA: The vision therapy described above exposed to me obvious brain alterations that were** *shocking* **to see—all signs of a damaged brain—whether by stroke or vascular dementia. He can't put numbers correctly on a clock face, or parts of the body in the right place... and Dale taught anatomy. This shocked my system so badly that I unconsciously totally repressed it; I had not been able to deal with it in Dale's presence during the session. Consequently, two years later (after Dale had passed) when a dear friend was showing me her four-year-old grandchild's drawings (which looked**

similar *but better than those drawings of Dale's for vision therapy*), I uncontrollably burst into tears and sobs as that scene all came rushing back to the surface. That emotional release happened nine months after Dale had died and yet was as fresh as the day it happened. You just never know when unresolved emotions will surface, and <u>I encourage you to deal with them as they come up and to get help as needed.</u>

5/16/2017 My Second Update to Doctors

Our family decision was made to not put Dale on Zoloft, although the prescription was written for it. In addition to the difficult history Dale has had with medications, I am extremely leery of giving him anything new based on his history of opiate addiction as well as the adverse and sometimes opposite (paradoxical) effects of prescription sleeping meds that caused great unrest and trauma during the early months after his massive stroke. I don't know if you saw it in his medical records, but when they were trying to get him able to sleep, we went through a number of medications, most of which caused adverse reactions; he was up most of the might, went days with hardly any rest, and ended up in a Posey bed. It was VERY traumatic for all of us and I do not EVER want to bring him to where he has to go through that kind of hell again. The only med that gave him rest was Seroquel, an antipsychotic. He stayed on it for nineteen months, including the five months it took to wean him off of it. Right now, he's not easily evaluating himself and doesn't give me many messages about how he's feeling, so my personal, continual observation is basically what we have to go on.

Our family opted to work with the natural process of adjusting melatonin. Dale's anxiety lessened with the melatonin adjustment, but episodes of anger and hatefulness continued at least one to two times daily for another week and the third time resulted in him walking away in anger, once in an unfamiliar place with traffic. It was awful. (NOTE: as a result of that experience, Dale no longer rode in the front passenger seat, but behind it with the child lock engaged, which also gave him no opportunity to touch the gear shift.)

At our aphasia support group meeting, I discussed this behavior with other caregivers and, among other suggestions, cannabis oil/CBD without the THC was brought up as having been successful for a few in the group. I pursued that with some research and determined it was worth a try. So, I've been administering three drops, about 10mg of CBD oil, since May 2nd and he has had no more episodes of anger/hatefulness since then. It has been two full weeks. I have been closely observing how it affects him and have given it around 8:00 a.m. along with other meds. It's been very helpful and seems to take twenty to thirty minutes to fully affect any anxiety if it has already surfaced, so I've determined to try and head it off. (I have also taken a dose myself to see what he might experience and found nothing noticeable, however I was not in an anxiety-producing situation, so the physiology was obviously different.) Dale's focus and therapy, communication, and humor have remained the same. Of course, there are still times of frustration, but if I notice anxiety building, I have given him another drop later in the day.

6/9/2017 My Third Update For Doctors

(Note to reader: these updates continue to be very specific and effective in describing behaviors and circumstances so they can serve as a conversation between me and the doctor without Dale having to hear details and concerns.)

    -Dale has had melatonin with a dose of CBD oil nightly, mostly 3mg melatonin

    -he's been waking at 4:30 a.m. even with an increase of melatonin or CBD oil or what time I administer them; I've varied about an hour.

-his sleep is good from about 10:30 p.m. - 4:30 a.m., although he'll still get up to use the bathroom a couple of times; then he either wakes up agitated and roams around for about half an hour or organizes his nightstand or continues to wake up every forty-five to sixty minutes or so and is unsettled even if I simply turn over in bed. At this point, there is no option for me to sleep in another room as I need to keep track of what he does, and he will search for me if I'm not there.

-I feel that if I give him the 5mg melatonin even alternating with the 3mg, then I've had more trouble discerning what causes any daytime agitation. (Increased daytime agitation is why we initiated CBD). However, right now I seem to think that he's just been experiencing more agitation during the day regardless of the melatonin dose, so I'm ready to alternate again.

-Dale's brain energy definitely gets depleted by all the various stimulation he is exposed to, and yet he wants to do things and be new places and watch a movie or a ball game, all of which can be quite a drain on him even if he's not the one being physically active. He's also now **much** more affected by heat/temperature.

-we drive to Sarasota a couple of times a week (forty-five minutes) for Dale's therapy and have been driving to Tampa once a week. This in itself has to be handled carefully because since he can't drive, just him sitting without being able to do anything at all can be anxiety-producing. We do listen to audiobooks and favorite music which normally helps and sometimes he will use a speech app on his iPad. However, the constant change in scenery, the refocusing outside the car, and awareness of traffic/weather and lights if we're out in the evening are factors with which he inadvertently has to contend.

-last night (6/8/17) for the first time in over six months, I gave him a tiny dose of Seroquel, .625mg – ¼ of a 25mg. tablet. He'd been on that for sleep for a year and a half after his first stroke but had been weaned off since June 2016 (had only used occasionally when traveling or in different time zones). So, last night he slept well, having had Seroquel plus 3mg melatonin plus the CBD dose. He woke up a bit groggy in the morning (but did **not** wake up agitated at 4:30 a.m.). I expect to use this for about a week in hopes of breaking that wake cycle and because we are staying in a hotel in Tampa while he attends an intensive speech program at USF so we'll be near the venue and have no back and forth daily driving.

6/11/2017 Ups and Downs

Upside: Dale gains so much encouragement from the Suncoast Aphasia Support Group, especially through the interactions at weekly reading groups. These wonderful folks have become our friends and Dale brightens up when he knows we'll be seeing them. In addition, several from the group have attended a semester of free classes for aphasics at USF in Tampa, and it has been our pleasure to ride up there with another attending couple. The interaction with teachers and students is outstanding and all are thriving.

Downside: We recognize that Dale is affected by vascular dementia from the stroke and his life is slowly changing, thus mine as well. We are engaged in using CBD (w/o THC) to assist Dale with anxiety and the results have been positive, although it is really a trial and error for us since dosing is subjective and Dale is not able to self-evaluate. *All calming is most welcome.*

I am again aware that I am not in control. I need to hear from You, Lord, "Calm in the storm, balm to the torn. When all else fails, You are true!"

6/26/2017 Helpful Hints

Listened to several of Teepa Snow's videos on dementia, noting that parts of the brain simply aren't working. Many of her helpful hints can apply to our situation. Her website states that Teepa's life mission is to shed a positive light on dementia. I highly suggest watching her videos on YouTube (see Appendix One).

Purposeful activities:
- load laundry
- put in and out of dryer
- take out forks and napkins
- fill dinner plate (unbreakable)
- move to music - dance or march
- put away silverware
- hang towel
- hang walking clothes

As for me, in the past couple of days, I was reminded to stop wasting my time with internet, apps, and games. Although these are escapes for me, it is counterproductive to be affected by the blue light emanating from the close devices in the evening. I'll be considering what I can do to replace this while Dale watches show or movies, some of which are of little interest to me, or we've seen multiple times. Lord, help me hear You for balance and use of all my time, including evening wind down. I was also reminded to revisit humor DAILY such as shows, jokes, or funny anecdotes.

7/4/2017 Doctor Report

It was an interesting week as I listened, changed, watched, hoped, and waited... how I need you, Lord.

Leukoaraiosis - term I noticed for the first time on recent neurologist's report. Actually, when I went back for comparison, I found it was on the report from January 2016, yet new to me now. Dale had some white matter show on his initial 2013 brain MRI;

ischemia intensified it, and memory is affected. It makes me so sad; it is difficult to note these factual findings. I have to cast these cares on the Lord and not carry them myself, fully trusting God to heal Dale in the present and give me grace and wisdom in the waiting.

Dale has occasionally felt unsettled in his stomach and wanted to talk about doctors. So, we are scheduled with his neurologist again at end of month for a quick update and talk with me. We will schedule with cardiologist as well; it's been over a year for both.

In the midst of any concern/questioning, there is always encouragement and blessing:
7/1 - Dale generated and clearly said "barbershop," a term we really don't use as we speak of the place by name, but it was perfect for his need! He smiled broadly as he heard himself and we rejoiced!
7/3 - received a call from the Chicago hotel where we'll be staying. They will transport us from the airport which is above and beyond their services and our requests! Thank you, God, for Your favor and for going before us.
-and, since changing Dale's night CBD dosage, he has slept well and awakened early, been clear-headed, and been somewhat more emotional, yet balanced.

Additionally, I am learning to be aware of even the smallest of mundane and familiar things. I serve as the sentinel for both of us and my perception/discernment of details and energy output is of utmost importance for the peace and safety of us both.

NOTE: Four years later as I write this in book form, it is SO hard for me to read the entries of these past six months. Vascular dementia kicked in surprisingly fast and I was unprepared to notice the signs and to recognize the timeline. Hindsight is so enlightening and that is one of the main reasons for this book and why I freely share these hard things. In the midst of living those months,

revelation and connections about behavior were slow in coming (I was often on overload myself). Now as I revisit this time, my prayer is that these entries will bring to light situations that will help the readers be better aware and prepared for their caregiving situations.

> *I serve as the sentinel for both of us and my perception/discernment of details and energy output is of utmost importance for the peace and safety of us both.*

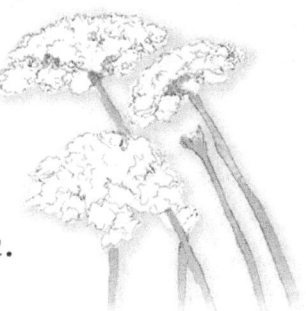

7/11/2017 Chicago Trip

The good, the facts, and the ugly. Sharing this in hopes that others can learn from even small details.

The good:
We went to Chicago accompanied, thankfully, by my sister Carol, for brain and vision therapy appointments with the two cutting-edge doctors: Dr. Donalee Markus, a cognitive restructuring specialist (see Appendix One), and a colleague Dr. Deborah Zelinsky (see Appendix One), an optometrist specializing in neural optometric rehabilitation. The appointments were wonderful, Dale appreciated the doctors, was comfortable working with them and navigated the offices well with few exceptions. They sent us to two other practitioners who work with brain/body trauma for calming and holistic rehab. Carol and I learned vast amounts of information and will implement all we can as soon as possible. Overall, we made the most of our trip while still moving at Dale's pace.

The facts:
Prior to the Chicago trip, I wrote this letter to my kids and inner circle of counsel and now share that personal email here along with any new observations noted for the doctors (that were additional to the previous Doctor Updates).

> *Dearest and closest to my heart,*
>
> *I've mentioned to you that I've been writing down observations re: dad for doctors, actually since April but in more detail while preparing for Chicago. Lin also asked me lots of details recently as well. And I've also reviewed many of dad's doctors' reports and looked up terminology as needed. Got some suggestions from Sam to have a doctor who explains well tell me the process of post-infarct (stroke) evolution. I expect to do that with Dad's neurologist the end of this month but may end up talking with Dr. Markus in Chicago.*
>
> *I'm attaching my notes just compiled Thursday; some changes are relatively new and some may be due to the many schedule changes this month and the effects of the intensive speech program; I know I've been affected by that effort and focus.* **This is emotional and I encourage you to truly give it to God; don't hold back or harden your heart. He knows the thoughts and intentions of your heart, and truth sets us free because the enemy is disarmed. I've recently learned that we try to shove uncomfortable thoughts away and that is why the Word warns us not to harden our hearts. By bringing thoughts to God, instead of holding them in darkness (that being the enemy's realm), Truth can predominate; these thoughts are brought into the light, and we are liberated.**

Most of the things I've noted line up with symptoms for **vascular dementia**, *caused by blood/ oxygen supply cut off to the brain by stroke. It is noteworthy that this form of dementia can improve or be slowed, specifically with good sleep, routine, and aerobic exercise. Those will be the areas I will focus our efforts on once we regroup after Chicago.*

We can talk about this now that you'll have this information anytime. Your insights and counsel are vital to us both and we thank God for you all. Love always, Mom

The following are my personal observations (dated 7/2/2017) that I gathered and sent to Chicago doctors to assist them in assessing Dale's needs. I also sent these doctors Dale's personal info and his Quantitative EEG report.

-Dale has a great sense of humor, thankfully, but also gets down on his situation and needs to be buoyed up by truth and perspective. He loves his family and wants to be involved in **everything**. We have had many people live with us over the years and, now that we've lived alone since this February, he often looks for others in the house.

-we walk or pool walk daily, sometimes bike ride on his recumbent trike, and workout in the gym (with a personal trainer) twice a week. Other than that, he is quite sedentary, and I wish that weren't so. Dale rarely initiates an activity or states what he'd like to do. We capitalize on that when it happens, but for the most part, he wants direction and doesn't do well with making decisions. It is difficult to find active things for him to do, especially with his own sports restrictions due to four joint replacements.

-Dale is now extremely sensitive to touch, and never used to be pre-stroke; he was tough. Now, I can't even go to hold his hand without him flinching and accusing me of hurting him. However, he can initiate touch and will be fine. This does seem to be more with me than with medical personnel or grandchildren so there may be more to it, but I don't know.

-often, he will talk to me while looking in a totally different direction or room. Can no longer always follow my voice to find me. Has been affected by low light for years and it is more evident since strokes that he needs well-lit spaces.

-(info re: our move to a new home and anger/hatefulness episodes, toileting issues, eating changes will *not be repeated here for the reader since they are all noted in earlier entries*)

-his attention in speech and vision therapies is good for forty-five-to-fifty-minute session and he can watch a familiar movie or show that is very interesting to him, however he is easily distracted, restless and wandering if something doesn't hold his attention. He can no longer tolerate watching intricate mysteries or stories that move too quickly, or are emotionally violent; he will stop them.

-Dale is capable of fine motor skills and, in the past four months, has been doing some art therapy and is able to button shirts and jeans (and chooses to wear those clothes), but he still can't coordinate instruction with response such as touching forefinger to thumb, even if he sees it modeled. He has been recovering his guitar skills for two years by playing with a friend weekly and muscle memory is an asset .

-he responds well to those with expertise (and uniforms of any sort) but doesn't usually want ME to teach or instruct him. The only exception is for his vocal therapy warmups which he is glad to do with me.

-Dale will gladly listen to audiobooks in the car or Talking Books at home. However at this point these only hold his attention for twenty to thirty minutes. It used to be longer, but now seems like it can get overwhelming, or he gets restless. His comprehension of the material is good, and he responds appropriately in the moment, but he can walk away from a book (or movie/show) without turning it off and not realize or care that he's missed the continuity.

-He is very social and freely interacts in conversation with others. In the past few months, his personal confidence in communicating has increased as he realized he can get his point across with effort and patience. However, this has provoked him to chatter on and on, assuming he'll be understood. This is difficult for me to explain to him.

-Dale knows all friends and family members by name but cannot always bring that name to the surface. He loves being with them, happy just actively watching and listening.

.-I also sent these doctors Dale's personal info and his quantitative EEG report.

The ugly:
Dale had a very rough time on the flight to Chicago. This following letter describes it to the doctors we had gone to visit so they would be aware but also asking for advice for the flight home.

> *Our flight today was delayed several times and we did not get to travel as I had hoped, earlier in before Dale got tired. Consequently, he became overwhelmed in the plane about an hour from landing in Chicago—tired, cramped space, noisy, bored, having no control of the situation and no understanding/reason. He was out of control, walking around, belligerent, and hateful. We've had some times like this before but never in an enclosed space like a plane; he was very close to be Tasered by an attendant. He was refusing to take anything I gave him, but I was finally able to get him to drink some juice with CBD oil in it and then take a small dose of Seroquel (which we normally use as a sleep aid), but that was not a quick fix.*
>
> *I expect with rest and balanced days while here; he will not be in that mode, but obviously I don't know for sure. What I do know is that I need a better plan of action to calm him*

before we make our next flight on Friday morning. I have no prescription for anything other than Seroquel. We have had success for the past month with CBD oil but are still adjusting dosages.

Any advice you can give will help. I plan to call his neurologist in the morning, but he hasn't seen Dale in a year (we have an appt on July 26th). I need to get him home safely on Friday and Florida is a long trip.

FOLLOW UP NOTE TO CHICAGO DOCTORS: Thankfully, our return trip home was successful with Dale only experiencing anxiety on descent due to great pain from the air pressure change (others were quite affected as well). Since he can't intentionally blow his nose or yawn to help get relief and doesn't grasp what is going on in the moment, he was quite distressed. I had upped his CBD dosing a lot and given him 31.25mg Seroquel. Thank you for helping us determine what to do for him.

Chapter Thirteen

HOW QUICKLY THINGS CHANGE

10/23/2017 Trauma

The following notes were written as an overview to update Dale's primary care doctor on the progression of anxiety he experienced from April through early August, some of which is noted above. Hindsight gives us amazing perspective and I share these with readers in hope that you can gain insight from our experiences. Most importantly, as I reviewed these three and four years later, it is obvious that the air travel highly affected Dale in ways we could not have imagined and of which <u>**we were not forewarned**</u>. Realizing that every individual has unique physical, medical, emotional, and mental factors, there is no blame for these happenings, simply regret that I and my family did not know more at the time. Our hope, and Dale's, was that these wonderful, expert doctors would provide additional therapeutic options for Dale's vision, speech, and brain health. And, gratefully, they did so very well. However, factors of which we were unaware and still cannot enumerate highly affected his anxiety responses in the following weeks, the outcome of which led to hospitalization in a behavioral facility, which with his poor communication and understanding had MANY negative effects. It is so very grieving for us all.

When we saw Dale's neurologist on 7/26, he prescribed Xanax and Effexor. <u>**Dale's response to Xanax was horrific, adverse, and paradoxical;**</u> we changed to Ativan after three days. By the end of the week, Dale had been *continually* anxious, agitated, and hateful which had caused me to call 911 three times. He would settle with the presence of uniformed personnel and then calmed when he allowed me to administer Seroquel.

This led to the 911 personnel suggesting Dale go to the ER, to which he finally agreed on 8/4 at 7:00 a.m. <u>**This began a horrific chain of events. I've learned I would sedate him myself than ever again put him and us through this unbelievable chain of events**</u>:

    -ER is not prepared to deal with a strong physical person with such poor understanding. Dale was highly overmedicated to keep him on the gurney until medically cleared to be transferred **six hours later** at 1:00 p.m.

    -since he lacked understanding and was (unintentionally) dangerous to himself and others, they invoked the Baker Act which then required Dale to be hospitalized in a facility.

    -the only behavioral unit with a bed available was nearly two hours away. They could not rouse him for transport due to heavy sedation.

    -this facility accepted him because they had a bed, but I was told days later *they were not suited to deal with geriatrics*; trauma had already begun with much medication

    -after he fainted *while I was visiting*, they moved him to a medical floor for evaluation, but it was not suited to his mental needs and consequently they put him under physical restraints while they evaluated his heart.

    -with this, he was not toileted and had to be fed by a staffer. **I was undone, furious and sobbing in the hall. They eventually called security to remove me from the area** (I did not fight them but did continue to explain the situation)

    -afterwards, while he on his regular floor, I could only visit him during visiting hours but spoke by phone to floor personnel several times a day

    -met with the head nurse and requested a conference with director and case manager *who wanted to* **send him home**

with me <u>***because they were not suited for his needs***</u>***!*** I claimed **UNSAFE DISCHARGE,** so they conceded to continue to treat him until they balanced his meds to quell the anxious and dangerous behavioral response.

Eleven days after going to the ER, after tremendous trauma to us both, and with him having an entire cocktail of meds, David and I brought him home (medicated on Geodon) to recover. My sister Carol stayed with us. Dale could hardly feed himself, find the toilet, talk, or engage in anything. My goal and that of my family was REST, PEACE, and ROUTINE. Fortunately we had wonderful, helpful advice from home health, along with PT and SLP. Carol and I were able to find a quality adult day care nearby, a safe place Dale could spend time with loving caregivers and several other adults who needed 24/7 assistance. This gave me respite for a few hours several days a week and Dale had the opportunity to socialize and interact with others, helping his recovery.

He's now been home for two months and we have been stabilized, although **Dale had marked decline in many areas as a result of this extended trauma.** I can only move forward slowly.

    -Dale has been peaceable since mid-September with Seroquel 50mg in the morning and 75mg accompanied by CBD oil in the evenings. This is very effective in calming. He no longer gets up multiple times during the night to use the bathroom, so we are both getting good sleep. He sleeps eleven to twelve hours and still takes Melatonin.

    -His neurologist had appts with him on 8/18 and 9/18 and is scheduled to see him again next week. *He and his staff were <u>amazingly</u> attentive to help us throughout this time, taking my calls whenever needed.* He expects in time we will see this as "a bump in the road." I hope so.

-He attends an adult day care center two days a week for four hours and is happy there. He gets safe, loving care and socialization and I have a few hours of respite.

-Dale needs constant supervision and assistance with dressing as well as direction for personal hygiene and eating. He eats whatever I prepare and cut up for him and uses special plates and utensils to assist him. Once he begins the showering process and I check the water temp, he showers/dries himself automatically.

-Dale seldom initiates activity but enjoys doing many things. We walk daily and he loves to sing and dance.

-He now engages in watching movies and sports and does well with family visits.

-Overstimulation is something that I have to watch for ALL THE TIME. He still has mood swings—sad, frustrated—and perseverates with OCD behavior about once a day, tires easily and gets more confused when tired or overstimulated.

INTERESTING SIDENOTE: *In the midst of Dale's restabilization, Hurricane Irma hit southwest Florida on September 10th.* **Upon learning that it was a wind storm, not a flood storm, and knowing that Dale would be anxiety-ridden in bumper-to-bumper evacuation traffic, we, the family, decided to weather the storm at home. Having plenty of provisions and home hurricane protection and making a "safe room" in our large walk-in closet, when the power went out at 7:00 p.m., I gave him his meds and we went to bed. Thankfully, it was over by the time he awakened, and David arrived with a generator as planned by 9:00 a.m. Our power was back on by noon and Dale was oblivious to anything further. SO glad our family has weathered many of these storms and were prepared to work together for our peace and safety.**

11/11/2017 Respite for Me

I realized today that I haven't journaled much personally. It has been very sporadic, mostly medical updates. I'm OK with that; it's just a revelation. I pray much, talk with God continually, listen, and pray with/for Dale. Writing is usually helpful for me, but so is REST.

I had the privilege of going to a cousin's wedding with Christy, David, and Steph. What a blessing to be "off duty"! So thankful for the caregivers at adult day care for going above and beyond to give me this day of respite. And what a joy to celebrate with family. Thank you, Lord.

12/17/2017 Medical Marijuana (MM)

We've been on a new path with medical marijuana oils since 11/30 when Dale received his MM ID card. Although I am at peace with moving into this realm, I am not used to being "in charge" of dosing without relying on doctor's advice along with my observations. And post-trauma Dale is not self-assessing at all. I have felt uncertainty—waffling, guesswork—in these few weeks and have realized that since God allowed me to be in this caregiving position, He will give me ALL I need to accomplish His purposes. I simply need to WAIT ON/ YIELD TO HIM. I have repented of lack of focus on Him, time wasted on other, mindless things, and have asked Holy Spirit's guidance to hear, wait and DO "God things", not simply "good things" - to follow and obey. This caregiving life is constant surrender to Him; *shouldn't all life be??*

We have dear family friends who are such an encouragement in their continual example of waiting on God's timing. Thank you for that example, Lord, and for my friend and neighbor's sweet reminder again to slow down and simplify.

12/21/2017 The "Lonely" Life

For these last months, I have basically been socially alone and often housebound. I pondered recently the 'lonely' life with just Jesus and me. It is a reality in many place and situations, and the way of most over history such as desert dwellers, pioneers, rural isolation, shepherds, explorers, even cave men. They provide good examples to follow. And, of course, Jesus... abandoned by even His closest.

Also encouraged by Joyce Meyer today to refuse and reject the enemy and his thoughts and plans immediately - at first notice! I will practice that! Let me state that I am not depressed but definitely feeling the lack of social interaction.

1/1/2018 Reflections on 2017

Since the last entry of mid-April, we've had many challenges. Summer was tough for a variety of reasons, although we learned much and met some amazing doctors and therapists who poured their expertise and kindness into both our lives.

Anxiety plagued Dale, worsening over several months, indicative of the progression of vascular dementia from his stroke and brain trauma. The anxiety medication that was prescribed by our trusted medical team to help him actually had a paradoxical effect and, in August, he was hospitalized for twelve days in order to regulate his medication and stabilize his system. He came home very fragile and traumatized and on six new meds; I needed help, my family needed help, and once again, God brought miraculous answers and connected me/us with individuals and associations perfectly matched to our needs.

Two weeks after he returned home, Hurricane Irma hit our coast bringing us new challenges. With prayer, the counsel of our kids, and past experience, we remained home, prepared with a safe room, supplies, medication, and family nearby... and all was well.

Within a month of returning home, Dale had decreased to one new medication, resumed PT and speech therapy at home, and attended a day center twice a week for his socialization and my respite. By December, he had comfortably found his role at the day center, leading dance, greeting and encouraging others, and showing his protective side when needed.

For Dale's restoration and healing, we walk through every open door. In May, we began using CBD oil, a cannabis product that brought a measure of calm. I continued to learn more about medical marijuana and Florida state approvals. By November, with the blessing of his primary care physician and neurologist, Dale received compassionate cannabis certification. Since the first of December he has been taking CBD oils with some THC. It's a very subjective process, since he doesn't self-assess, and the total observation/evaluation is mine. Results are that his peace is now constant, he has improved engagement, fewer times of overstimulation, and day meds have been cut by 75% as of this week. Our family is pleased and look forward to increased clarity as Dale continues this adjustment.

We continue to realize the value of safe walking and community in our lives.

SAFE WALKING:
...in the physical:
-a new home with opportunities to get out and walk in the fresh air and sunshine usually twice a day on safe streets and sidewalks,
-the opportunity to walk through a serious medical situation and to overcome a setback
-a continual walk toward restoration and health

-making strides in gaining knowledge daily in many varied areas
...in the spiritual:
-God's faithfulness in leading our steps is UNFAILING. Oh, how I need Him for safe walking each day. At times, when I'm distracted and caught up in situations, I tend to react. But when I take time to pause, waiting to hear how to respond, not react, God provides the next step, all I need: Light for the path, Daily Bread.

COMMUNITY:

-Since Dale's first stroke three years ago, we've gathered a team around us for counsel and support, some for a short season, others continuous, yet always changing, fluid and bringing life: family, some are new friends, some medical or therapists - our community.

-We are made for community, patterned after the perfection of the Trinity, the oneness of Father, Son/Jesus, and Holy Spirit. Everyone can function at their best in community as they give and receive, meet needs, and together face opportunities and challenges for growth, intimacy, and authenticity.

-Our families are our community. We are blessed to have our son David and his family just a few minutes away, our daughter Christy just 1½ hours away, and Dale's sister, my brother, and their spouses only an hour down the highway, affording us physical visits where we can hug and 'reach out and touch' one another.

-The blessing of technology allows us to talk with or FaceTime our daughter in CA, sisters in Tallahassee, OH, and AZ, numerous extended family, and even our career military nephew overseas

-In our new neighborhood, we can walk down the street, connecting by just stopping to talk with other walkers, or those on their porches, working in the yard or playing tennis. There's a whole new community here and we are grateful to be here, to relate, to be welcomed and to have a part in the lives of others.

-Our support groups, churches, and friends everywhere are all our community. Oh, how we need each other!

Dale and I miss the community life that used to be a vital part of our everyday world (sometimes desperately). Our life has changed:

- phone calls are no longer spontaneous,
- some friends weren't able to cope with the changes in Dale/our lifestyle and we no longer see them,
- we presently don't yet travel over forty-five minutes by car
- expectations have been altered to Dale's capacity
- grace has become more important

Our focus is not holding on to what <u>was</u>,
so we can embrace WHAT IS.

I'll close with thoughts recently sent to me that you might consider them as well:

We are made for community and to experience its goodness.
We need it. You need it. I need it.

Find a way to echo God's lovingkindness day's end:

- Light a candle
- Speak a blessing over someone
- Simply listen
- Leave a love note on a pillow
- Send a goodnight text
- Read a devotional out loud
- Hold that hug
- Share a YouTube worship song
- Share a cup of warm tea and cookies

Chapter Fourteen

HOMEBOUND

1/30/2018 Soul Food

Much change continues. After two months on medical marijuana management, Dale is clearer and being weaned from Seroquel. I am slowly moving step by step, needing Holy Spirit for discernment, observation, and wisdom. He is faithful and I am where I need to be; at His feet, yielded and listening. We are living the simple life; a quiet, peaceful, routine, good sleep, good food, therapy at home, daily walking, contact with loved ones daily, simple social times.

Both of us have gleaned much from Bill Johnson sermons and Joyce Meyer. That is where we are "fed" now along with Matthew, John, and Acts videos, *Streams in the Desert,* and personal encouragement from the Body of Christ. Dale is engaged and we "discuss" as we can, always answering his questions.

Personally, I listen to/read the Gospels regularly to know Jesus better. "<u>The Lord IS MY Shepherd,</u> and I <u>shall NOT WANT</u> (lack)." I speak this ALOUD whenever the enemy raises concerns about not being shepherded/cared for or needing something. All is well.

2/4/2018 His Keeping Power

Thank you, Lord, for keeping me... in the midst of sorrow, temptation to self-pity, whining, pining, or envy. YOU faithfully present TRUTH and insights into Your plan. I am Yours, available to be broken to be used, not a foreign concept. Seeds are broken open for a plant to come forth; grains are broken or crushed to be used as flour for bread and food.

Holy Spirit, keep me mindful to turn my heart and incline my ear to You at each wrenching of my heart, to pray for neighbors, loved ones, the hurting, neglected, abused, cast aside, or forgotten. Thank You for building Your compassion in me. Lead on and I follow...

3/17/2018 The Grieving is Real

I SO wanted to journal yesterday, to pour out my heart, filled with tears and need. The Lord IS my shepherd and my husband - hallelujah! I praise Him in/for that Truth when I "feel" husbandless and shepherdless in the physical. It hurts and I wrestle with self-pity. O God, I know David poured out his heart to You honestly in the Psalms and You provided those writings for us to know. I cry to You, Lord. <u>You ARE MY</u> Shepherd and I <u>DO NOT LACK</u> anything truly needed. You ARE my Strength and my Song. When (not if) my heart is overwhelmed, lead me to the Rock that is higher than I.

The grieving is real. Yet, because of Jesus, I do not grieve without Hope. The loss is great, but I do not want, for You are with me, Lord, Your rod and staff, they comfort me, guiding, protecting, keeping me on Your path for my life, whatever that looks like. The other day I cried, "I don't want to be an inspiration!" This life is hard, lonely, painful, sacrificial, filled with unknown. But I'm not moved by what I feel, I'm just moved by the Word of God. More of me dies daily. So be it, Lord, consume me, everything that does not look like You. And there has been much lately, when hard-pressed, the ugly has come out. I repent, Lord, and direct my eyes to You, the Author and Finisher of my faith. Complete Your work in me, Lord. Create in me a clean heart and renew a right spirit within me. I trust in You and praise Your Holy Name.

5/7/2018 Thankful For Caring Bridge

Well, here I am again and so grateful for this blog site. It is easy to spend much time repeating myself in text or conversation, so I have once again turned to Caring Bridge to connect with those who need to know and/or care.

Things have changed with Dale this week. After much reflection and conversation yesterday, it appears that Dale had another stroke last Saturday. He was awakened in the night by a short cough, yet one that caused him to momentarily gasp for breath; he awoke startled and scared. I was able to calm him and start some treatment and he slept well all night. However, when he awoke in the morning and went to the bathroom, on his way back to bed he collapsed against the dresser and to the floor. I saw this from the other side of the room and sat with him on the floor to evaluate. With Dale's "normal" condition of aphasia and difficulty following instructions, there were no other specific indicators of stroke such as paralysis/droop, lack of recognition, etc. I attributed the fall to low blood sugar, sleepiness, or getting up too quickly. I slowly got him back to bed. He slept much of the day and by late afternoon, a bruise appeared on his right side ribs under his arm from the fall. This caused him much discomfort over the next few days, and he was battling the congestion/cough; a few nights he was up and down for hours. He slept long and did little physically during the week, which I attributed to his physical issues.

> **NOTE: An aside here...from what we later learned, this may not have been a stroke, but part of the syndrome that we learned about in July. Regardless, our family has agreed to care for Dale at home as much as possible. Hospitals, and sometimes doctors' offices, quickly become traumatic because he doesn't speak clearly and is more confused when he's upset by unfamiliar or**

anxious circumstances; this quickly escalates to a situation that is bad for Dale all around, and difficult for medical personnel and family. **Peace and safety for all is a priority.**

So, now we're just over a week after the fall and yesterday/Monday was totally NOT normal... not even our "normal," starting with he was hardly able to make it home on our typical morning neighborhood walk. He had low blood pressure when I was able to check it, and that's after coffee and breakfast. I became very observant, talked with our decision "team" consisting of family and primary care and by evening, recounted the many things that had changed during the week, all of which point to a stroke/TIA event and all of which were masked by congestion and pain from the bruised ribs. He had a long night's sleep, resting for twelve to thirteen hours, poor appetite, difficulty locating me by my voice, vision issues such as not seeing lower quadrant including the toilet, and, for the past two days, bumping into things lower than his knees.

Peace and safety for all is a priority.

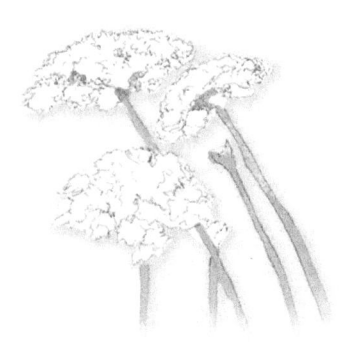

I talked with the nurse again at the end of day yesterday and expect to get him to our doctor today for assessment and bloodwork, but they know he might not be able to do the lab. At that time, we'll check into home health, etc. Have already cleared our schedule so he can rest as needed in familiar, quiet surroundings and have all the meds/supplements he needs on hand, thankfully.

We are blessed with God's grace and strength and good counsel from family and medical team (our primary care doctor and nurse have known us for decades); just need prayer for peace, wisdom, and good rest for us both (your support, TLC, and food are welcome also).
It's 5:20 a.m. now and I've been up for two hours. I am not concerned and will catch up, simply using the time I'm awake to connect with you all.

5/8/2018 Settling In...

I don't plan to write often, but many hoped for an update:

We had a good night; Dale slept twelve hours. I began saturating his system with CBD and/or THC when he awoke at 3:00 a.m. and continued to do so every couple of hours throughout the day.

On morning walk after breakfast, he made it to three houses short of the block before energy depletion; it was sudden and confusing. I'll be adjusting our walks to back and forth down our street always within three houses from ours until I see his endurance increase. I'm also on the lookout for a loaner wheelchair should we need it.

The lab visit and doctor appointment went well; his BP is good, lungs clear, and no residual from congestion. Dale remains on Eliquis which thins blood and, although no med is PERFECT, it basically prevents clots from the heart. However, there are many other factors which could provoke stroke/TIA such as pieces of plaque breaking off in the arteries. Doctor couldn't confirm stroke without extensive tests, and maybe not even *with* tests (reminder: in 2014, they didn't know the cause of his massive stroke), and we're not putting Dale through another trauma of hospitalization/extensive testing. Also, vascular dementia is a factor brought on by the first/major stroke and will try to run its ugly course; God is the Restorer and that is in His hands. *My direction is to treat Dale as I would want to be treated, always foremost in my mind.* Got a prescription for home health; Dale can have whatever therapy is available at home in familiar surroundings.

So, we walked three times today with two outings and a little dancing, he said some good words and there was PEACE, we watched Stars Wars and he stayed engaged, and he ate well. I've started taking him by the hand and leading instead of telling him what direction or that dinner's ready which helps with much less confusion. I spoke with my friend who runs the adult day center, and she was very encouraging about home care. The goal is to keep him safe and comfortable, adjusting priorities as needed. Needs now that we are basically homebound:

- we have one volunteer to run errands in town
- need someone do a pickup for us in Venice
- wheelchair to borrow, hopefully lightweight

Many are praying for which we are thankful. One longtime friend called today to say I've been on her mind ALL week with a sense that prayer was needed. She had trouble locating my phone number and, in the meantime, saw my Facebook™ post and then knew why'd she been praying all week so called to encourage me/us that God is orchestrating help that's needed. I KNOW He is, and I trust Him. May His will be done on earth (that's in us...) as it is in Heaven.

5/15/2018 One Week Later...

Glad to say that Dale is greatly improved and basically back to his present "normal," including singing and dancing. With the exception of endurance/energy, he is doing everything as he had been... and even more! I'm measuring endurance right now by our daily walks. Previous to this episode, our normal walks were one to one-and-a-half miles morning and evening, so, when he couldn't make it around our .2-mile block, it was a significant difference. We pulled back and walked a short route more often, staying close to the house, four-five times a day, and within three-four days, he was fine walking the entire block. We increased by a house or two every time we could and this morning, he walked a half mile loop. I am grateful.

We've had several friends over for visits and Dale has been engaged comfortably for nearly two hours. Christy and my niece Lauren were here for Mother's Day afternoon and Dale only needed a short nap during that time. Yesterday he had three hour-long evaluations by home health therapists, was quite tired after each one, but he recovered after a short nap. We went to our grandson's awards presentation for about an hour Monday night; Dale did fine but was exhausted by all the stimulation of many moving around, much to watch, a dark auditorium, etc., especially at 7:00 p.m. when he is normally winding down. We'll have therapies here at the house for as long as they are approved by Medicare. The familiar surroundings and lack of distractions from others give him the opportunity to focus on the therapies alone. He hasn't had OT for several years, so I'm particularly pleased with that.

Good news bonus: in the past three days, Dale's had clearer speech, is more interested in saying words, initiates squats and tai chi type movements several times a day, even on walks. I attribute these improvements to increased CBD/THC for over a week now.

5/29/2018 Considering Future Changes

My "free" time is limited. Since it's been just the two of us, I only have windows of opportunity even to talk on the phone for business or pleasure considering that it's best not to discuss medical things in front of Dale. He doesn't usually realize I'm talking on the phone so will join in or interrupt. That being said, I am so grateful for those of you who connect here on Caring Bridge, leave messages, send notes, and pray for us. I just can't respond and wish I could... so I pray God's blessings on you and your families.

This facet of our life is *highly restricted* and certainly one we never would have chosen. Connection with the "outside world" is limited by what Dale can handle with his energy and emotions as well as by his time and priorities so there are now many things I'm not aware of, including current events and happenings in the lives of our friends. Those precious individuals who have been able to visit us are rays of sunshine in my life and those who help with various tasks are my *angels*. Bless them, Lord, as they give of themselves to us.

I have talked with family in the past few days as many changes are evident with Dale. He had a very rough night about a week ago and fell twice on his way back from the toilet; I brought out a wheelchair to transport him until the home health nurse arrived and we could check his strength. I'm writing of this because that is not at all normal and is definitely a red light that needs attention. Dale continues to sleep over twelve hours at night and still sleeps more after breakfast. Afternoons are his most engaged time, and he will walk short distances outside and do therapy comfortably but with a great expenditure of energy and needed recovery time. He's eating and drinking well and for that I am grateful. His cognition and attention span show decline and are noticeable.

Home and walking the neighborhood have recently become his entire world and even the grocery store has become too much stimulation and energy output. I've had others shop for me all this month; that is also why therapists are coming here to the house. It is very different. As a result, and after talking with family, I am engaging with others who have more experience in this caregiving arena so that I can obtain wise counsel for future decisions.

Our decisions to be made by two main factors:
1) Dale's personal wishes expressed when he still had all his mind about him, and 2) that we will treat him in the manner in which we would want to be treated if we were in his situation.

That is being stated so you know how to pray; we are not without hope; Jesus is Hope and He is with us. God is faithful to show me and us each next step. For that, I am most grateful. I trust Him implicitly. And in the face of so much change, I have been greatly encouraged today by the personal testimony of a friend who over a year ago asked us over to share about his miraculous healing after many years of horrific, unending pain and crippling joints, sitting in a chair not moving for hours on end. He is basically our age and is now recovered and functioning ably every day, ministering *around the world* to those in need, and wanting to use all the energy and ability he has. With that type of true healing experience in front of me, I want to clearly say that I know Jesus is our Healer and this could happen to Dale any day. *Our lives are in His hands.*

So, we move forward step by step. I am now using more of my alone time while Dale sleeps to pray for and encourage others in whatever way I can. To that end, I am thankful for technology available to contact others so quickly when time does permit. Each day is different and flexible, keeping me on my knees at Jesus' feet. *Where else should I be?*

> **NOTE: Over the next few weeks, I came to realize that this last episode in early May greatly affected other aspects of Dale's brain, thinking and behavior, in addition to whatever changes may have been provoked by vascular dementia.** *It is important for others facing this decline to realize that social and relational norms may no longer be normal.* **In fact, with Alzheimer's and dementia, it is typical for relational recognition to disappear (with**

the exception of disjointed lucid moments). There is so much about the brain that is unknown, and researchers can only record commonalities in behaviors for which families can be forewarned. Many families choose not to learn about these tragic changes, but I found learning from other's experiences softened the emotional blows that come with decline and change.

This *relational* change was blockbuster for all involved; Dale no longer understood marriage and family relationships, he only knew familiarity and who he trusted. Any male he recognized, he trusted; any female he knew could easily be a replacement for me! That was hard for all of us and caused a few surprising and awkward physical touches. Although this behavior is well-known with teachers and caregivers of exceptionally brain-affected individuals, it was new to me and our loved ones. VERY HARD yet needed to be discussed and we did so openly.

On July 10, our 47th anniversary: Dale could not understand the terms anniversary, marriage, wife, husband, child, etc. or how he and I fit into that realm. However, when I showed him our wedding pictures, he immediately brightened and could relate to us in that moment - young – yet didn't recognize his present self in pictures or know my relationship to him. He could still latch onto conversations for a short time as others initiated topics with which he retained attachment - fishing, sports, grandkids, names, God, food. I had much grieving over that loss and had not been prepared for it although it immediately made sense to me as I acknowledged all the other areas in which he had losses, especially meals and eating as well as toileting.

6/5/2018 This Is The Day that the Lord Has Made...

...let us rejoice and be glad in it...

Some days are SO much harder than others, those days with situations we honestly wish didn't have to be a part of our lives. *Yesterday was one of those days*, presenting new trials, emotions and complications that don't have easy answers. So, I run to the quiet, the beautiful, that I can be restored. I'm grateful to know The Answer, the One I can turn to anytime, anywhere, for any reason. He is our Refuge, our Refreshing, our Peace, our Joy, our Everything. Oh, how I need Him, how Dale needs Him, and I pray for Dale to sense God's presence, for his spirit to commune with Holy Spirit in ways that are far too mysterious for my understanding. Yet I know that we are spirit, soul, and body - eternal beings - and that the body is the clay, the ash, the temple for the eternal and, although the body is daily moving toward death, the spirit is alive and well.

Do you know Him? Jesus, the Messiah, God's Chosen to bring Life into this dying world? There is no other way to Eternal Life, life with God. Eternity is real, far more real than this physical world that takes up so much of our time and energy. Whether we acknowledge it or not, eternity IS. Whether we acknowledge God or not, He IS. We are small; He is great, majestic, the all-knowing Creator. With awe, we consider the vast marvels of technology, yet fall short in acknowledging the multitudinous wonders in the nature around us, that they are created by the Master Designer, wondrous to behold.

I was emotionally wiped out yesterday, but not defeated; sad, but not forlorn; stymied, but not without hope; at the end of myself, but not without knowing I just needed one next step to continue. He lights my path, even if the light simply goes as far as the next footfall. That's really all I need, my daily bread, manna from Heaven that brings Life.

I hesitate to share in this journal sometimes; it can be pretty raw. And then, unexpectedly, I'll receive a note that our journey has inspired someone to be strong in spirit and faith. After having told God, "I'm tired of being an inspiration," I repent of my selfishness, and over and over again yield to His plan to use me/us in whatever way serves Him and others best. He is the Potter; I am the clay. This lump of clay certainly doesn't claim to know what the Potter is making or His purpose; I choose to yield and let Him make me what He wills. I gain SO MUCH COURAGE AND INSIGHT from the writings of others who've gone through life's trials before me. How can I not openly share my life that others may be encouraged as well?

So, there you have it. I'll keep taking the days the Lord has made one step at a time, rejoicing in even the little things, looking up and encouraging you to do the same so we can bring Life to one another.

> *I gain so much courage and insight from the writings of others who've gone through life's trials before me. How can I not openly share my life that others may be encouraged as well?*

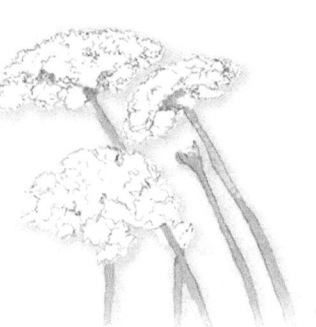

6/15/2018 Showers of Blessing

One of my parents' favorite songs that I consequently learned as a child was *April Showers*:

> "When the April showers, They come your way,
> They bring the flowers that bloom in May.
> So, keep on singing, have no regrets,
> Because it isn't raining rain, you know,

It's raining violets.
And when you see clouds up on the hill,
You soon will see crowds of daffodils.
So, keep on looking for the bluebird and listening for his song
Whenever April showers come along."

So, today's reading from the devotional *Streams in the Desert* struck a familiar chord with me; its truth is evident. Be blessed in the reading and take time to ponder.

> *He named the...child Ephraim... "God has **made me fruitful in the land of my suffering**.*   Genesis 41:52

"It isn't raining rain for you. It's raining blessing. For, if you will but believe your Father's Word, under that beating rain are springing up spiritual flowers of such fragrance and beauty as never before grew in that stormless, unchastened life of yours. You indeed see the rain. But do you see also the flowers? You are *pained by the testings*. But God sees the sweet flower of **faith** which is upspringing in your life under those very trials. You shrink from the suffering. But God sees the tender **compassion** for other sufferers which is finding birth in your soul. Your heart winces under the sore bereavement. But God sees the **deepening and enriching** which that sorrow has brought to you. It isn't raining afflictions for you. It is raining **tenderness, love, compassion, patience**, and a thousand other flowers and fruits of the blessed Spirit, which are bringing into your life such a **spiritual enrichment** as all the fullness of worldly prosperity and ease was never able to beget in your innermost soul." —J. M. McC[4]

---

[4] (Cowman, Streams in the Desert 1999)

7/2/2018 New Therapy Possibility?

Well, sometimes things move quickly! Saturday morning, a therapy option resurfaced as a possibility that I think Dale would want me to consider - Hyperbaric Oxygen Therapy (HBOT). I sent out feelers to several of "Team Dale" who were likely to have insights, and was encouraged to move forward, however, we didn't know at that point if he could actually handle the therapy or if it was available nearby.

Twenty-four hours later, Sunday morning, I had a conversation with the owner of a facility in Sarasota, the only one in the area with a multi-person chamber that we would need, and we began digging into this opportunity becoming a reality for Dale. I made a list of questions and contacted our trusted cohort, Sam, to do further research for me and to call the owner on my behalf with detailed questions. After helpful and informative conversation between owners and Sam in the evening, Sam sent me details with a positive "go ahead" to move forward unless a door closed.

This morning, Monday, I called the owner with my last questions and a request for a "dry run" tomorrow/Tuesday to run through dosing, travel, time away from home, and what we'd need to bring with us. It was agreed upon and we are at peace.

So, by faith, we are moving forward. Father has already provided a home for our friends to stay in while they help us. I was blessed and amazed at that gracious friend's hospitality. And these friends have received their own blessings of provision for the duration as well. I can only marvel at what God is putting together and trust Him for the rest of the needs. Dale can begin this Thursday and is scheduled to be in the chamber two hours daily for twenty-six to twenty-eight days straight so we expect to be driving to Sarasota nearly an hour away for all of July, thus my need for the help of others. Here are the prayer requests:

> -that we will be mindful of all the facets of this situation that affect Dale: transitions, correct dosing, quiet/down time, total time away from home
> -wisdom and discernment for us and staff during therapy
> -peace surrounding the entire process and duration
> -Dale's good sleep and easy morning waking and readying
> -comfortable, enjoyable, peaceful travel
> -Dale's understanding and smooth instruction-following to change into/out of scrubs for treatment
> -physical comfort (ears, eyes...) with air pressure changes
> -things to occupy him while in the HBOT chamber
> -my well-being and Sam's during this process
> -household needs for us and Sam's family this month
> -finances - this round is $7,000-8,000 all told plus gas.

To answer some questions, I'm including a link below. We know that some people continue with further rounds of therapy; we are taking this one step at a time. We also know that HBOT is standard procedure in Europe and Dale would already have had this with his condition had we lived there.

https://www.amenclinics.com/intensive-healing-for-your-brain/

Scan here for more information

7/6/2018 Facing the Hard Questions

Our 'dry run' at HBOT facility went well in many ways: travel, overall length of time away from home worked fine, Dale successfully saw many new people and places and tried many new things. The owners were warm, welcoming, knowledgeable and most accommodating - place we will definitely recommend. We came away ready to regroup and slow down the pace of acclimating Dale to the therapy, carefully and circumspectly considering each step and the timing.

APPARENTLY NOT TO HAPPEN.

The next morning, July 4th, Dale collapsed to the ground momentarily only a half block into our walk. Christy was with us, and we did our best to help him and then called a friend to bring the transport chair and wheeled him home. The rest of the day was low key at home and relaxed, with Dale only walking around inside the house. However, by the following morning, July 5th, Dale had collapsed four times in nine hours simply walking to the bathroom. *It was awful to witness, and we had no way of preventing it.* It was obvious he could sense it coming on but could do nothing to control it. They lasted only seconds and he'd crawl to the bed. It was scary, and I fell along with him once. It was only by the grace of God we both weren't hurt.

> **NOTE: Two new factors had surfaced:**
> -a phone conference with his doctor brought to light the possibility of Sick Sinus Syndrome in which the heart's natural pacemaker located in the right atrium becomes damaged and is no longer able to generate normal heartbeats at the normal rate.
> -Dale was bruising from the falls and likely had some internal bleeding as a result.
> Consequently, in honoring Dale's request for us not to treat anything further that would simply cause an extension of his present (or worsening) quality of life, AND to treat him as I/we would want others to treat us if we were in that situation, I made the decision, with my family's agreement, to take him off the blood thinner so he wouldn't hemorrhage internally from the increasing falls. We had already determined NOT to do any further

testing, even on his heart. His decline is obvious to us all and his peace, safety and comfort remain our priority.

Friends came to stay with us for safety. **Dale spent the next forty hours sleeping**, except for few intermittent wakings for toilet and liquids; *I spent it recognizing the realities in which I can't help him and considering with family the next step in his care.* **Very hard facing this and making decisions.** He awoke late this afternoon (forty-four hours later), revived and in great need of activity, movement, and food. He ate an entire solid meal and walked much around the house of his own accord, oblivious to danger.

Could he fall? Hurt himself? Yes. Could I stop that from happening? Could anyone or any facility stop that from happening? **NO, not without drugs or restraints.** *Is that how I would want to live - drugged, restrained? NO, again.* So, I determined to yield control and continue advising, cautioning, watching, praying, and giving NO place to fear... and family agreed.

And then there's GOD... this is no surprise to Him. So, we move forward, once again acknowledging our limitations and trusting God for His next step. **We can no longer live alone, the two of us.**
What's ahead? He's not yet ready for Hospice (I did have him evaluated for it). A care facility? Communal living? We are facing the great unknown once again. Again, I find myself on my knees at Jesus's feet, right where I belong. Where He leads me, I will follow.

Simply put, now you know our prayer needs. And we know we can't do this alone; your love and support bring life. Thank you for it.

7/13/2018 Adjusting...

It's been a week since Dale began to revive from his falling ordeal. Your prayers and support have been impactful during this time and our family thanks you. Since July 6th, Dale has continued to recover and his system is once again settling into a another "new normal," stabilizing and moving forward. He still has a big energy deficit but eating/sleeping well and engaging in activities/exercise/socializing. I have spoken with medical staff from Dale's primary care and neurologist as well as home health. All agree that the trauma of further testing is not in Dale's best interests (although I hope to have blood and urine retested as soon as home health is reinstated) and that we will proceed with home care, round-the-clock detailed observation, and treating symptoms for Dale's comfort and peace of mind; former HBOT plans are no longer on the table. *Wanted you all to know that this decision has been made and that Christy, David, and Stephanie are in agreement.*

That being said, as I wrote about our future on Caring Bridge last week, the words 'communal living' came to mind, and I wrote them down. I've never used that term in reference to our care before. To make a long story short, I slept on it, and it was on my mind several times during the night and again in the morning. I felt I should ask Sam and Cyndi Steen, our dear longtime friends/family to live with us as we are developing a communal living plan. The goal remains the same as stated before that Donna and Dale will not live simply as two any longer, that there will always be a third person in the house with anyone who is taking care of Dale so that if the primary caregiver for that day becomes incapacitated by accident or illness, there will be another 'body' in the house to make a phone call and sound the alarm. I envision the possibility of making a rotating schedule and a rotating calendar incorporating others who have volunteered as well as a private duty nurse to fill in so that each of us can have a full respite day at least once a week. We know other families with highly incapacitating needs who manage life and care with this kind of schedule. The Steens' commitment is to provide cohesion and consistency to see this communal living established, no timeline except God's. We know it takes time to establish routine, gather resources and train all those who God will bring in - both to live here with us and to volunteer for shifts.

We moved to Park Forest for community and safe walking: God is redefining that vision. For those of you who still want to come and stay with us, we have two neighbors who have already made their guest rooms available for our family and friends as needed!

FYI - when the term communal living first came to my mind, I was immediately reminded of Francis Schaeffer's L'Abri community that I have always admired, and also of the home mentioned at the end of *The Hiding Place*, Corrie ten Boom's sister's vision of a place for war refugees and concentration camp survivors to live in community for restoration and healing. I was later reminded of our friends in China who began with a small home facility that expanded into a five-story home and other buildings for single mothers and their children as well as elderly, all living in community.

So, as we draw aside to develop and establish all aspects of this communal living, I don't expect to journal much in Caring Bridge. Please pray for all of us involved in this process, including those who are still to become a part of it.

Chapter Fifteen

CHANGING ADDRESSES

8/1/2018 Never Wanted To Be At This Place

It's 9:11 p.m. and **I'm sitting in my bed alone beginning a whole new chapter of our lives.** After a very rough week of ups and downs with anxiety and adjusting doses for Dale, a conference with Christy and David last night culminated in us agreeing that **we could no longer safely and peaceably sustain life together at home even with help...** and <u>that we need to find the suitable place that God has for Dale's care.</u> Many tears. Lots of assurances. Sketchy plans to start things in motion for long term care, a process with which we are not familiar, calling his doctors in the morning for the process.

I slept little last night with Dale by my side. Not that I was worried; although my head was filled with many things, I was at peace. We are created as eternal beings, in the image of God. The spirit is forever; it's the body that fades and returns to dust. In Dale's case, his spirit will live on eternally with God as for decades he has believed in Jesus as God's Son and His atonement for our sins on the cross resulting in a restored relationship with God Himself. For months now, as Dale's mind has waned in comprehension, I've been reminded to speak to his spirit, to feed and exercise the eternal.

So, as God goes before us, this morning Dale awoke at 7:00 a.m. to toilet and fell once again as he returned to bed, not even able to pull himself up onto it this time. Sam and I struggled to help him and yet he was barely mindful of his need for assistance and proceeded to try to get off the bed and move about on his own. With help from some medication, he finally resettled and fell asleep. He awoke again at 10:00 a.m. to use the toilet, then again fell to the floor in the bathroom, scraping his back on the shower door and didn't get up - stunned although he remained conscious.

I called 911 while Sam attended him, Dale remaining on the floor with us in attendance. He was very subdued but responsive. He had no injuries, just cuts and scrapes, and received patient, conscientious care from the paramedics, then at North Port ER (as the closer Englewood Hospital was on CT scan deviation). Afterwards he was transported to Sarasota Memorial for three days of observation.

Thus, the Medicare process to move into long term care was started for us, nearly before I had a chance to make any phone calls. And glory to God, we normally would not have been transported to NPER, twenty-nine miles away, when ECH is two miles from our house. However, SMH is where all Dale's stroke care has been with all his records and his neurologist is there and, since NP is a branch of SMH, so that's where he was taken. I am most grateful.

I am also amazed and blessed by the caring, experienced professionals who presently are caring for Dale at SMH. We are likeminded in seeking peace and safety for Dale and they were putting feet to their words even before I left. I have every confidence that God is directing his care far better than I ever could.

So, I am writing this from my bed, alone. *Dale will not be returning to this house with the exception of a miracle*. Tomorrow, the process continues to find a home for Dale. We've already been blessed with several friends who are well-suited to advise us. Christy, David, and family are on board to help and the Steens are able to stay for a time to assist in helping me. Other family and friends are already giving us great support.

As always, your prayers are important to us. God is with us, His evidence surrounds us as we are led by Holy Spirit and walking in His peace. I'll post as decisions are made, but no daily reports on Dale as he is only under observation, not treatment.

> *I am writing this from my bed, alone. Dale will not be returning to this house with the exception of a miracle.*

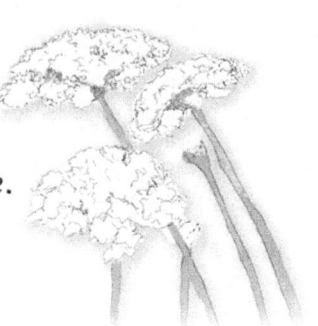

8/10/2018 God's Morning

We have just turned Dale over to Hospice. It appears he's had a massive stroke, is in the ER, not suffering but totally unresponsive. My sister Nancy is with me; the family is at peace, and I'm well cared for as we wait for transport to the Hospice House.

8/11/2018 Hospice House…

Long day. We are well and one of us is staying with Dale continually. He remains unresponsive. We are truly overwhelmed by prayers and notes from hundreds. Read many out loud to Dale, encouraging his spirit in your love and prayers for us all. Dale's room at Hospice is large and beautiful with a living area that enables us to comfortably have family and friends with him and us and a screened porch for fresh air and nature.

Dale continues to be nearly always at peace, except when they move or clean him... and they are SO gentle and honoring. Breathing has become more labored and uneven, with rattling sounds that tend to go right through me. This is very hard for me (and I've been wearing earplugs some or turning up the music). We all talk with him all the time and know He is near.

I went home along with my sister for a few hours this morning for breakfast and to swim, shower, and pack. Cyndi and Hope were here with Dale then; presence is important. We are not leaving him alone in his room. Kim and Kevin came for much of the day and got great comfort by being with Dale. Family had dinner here in the facility's big dining room. Christy's best school friend and college roommate came with her mother. It was a warm and welcome visit. Her dad, a Messianic Rabbi, has made himself available to us as pastor since ours has moved to Gainesville; he'll come over tomorrow. Christy's housemate arrived tonight, and they'll all stay overnight at David's. Then I had the pleasure (and distraction) of working with grandson Joshua, revising his application letters for his future after senior year.

So grateful Nancy is here with me and the Steens are handling the household.

8/14/2018 The Waiting...

Dale's body is still lingering but he is in Jesus's tender care and is at peace. I found an artist's rendering that is very close to the vision I had on August 1st of my releasing total control of Dale's care into the Lord's arms... only one set of footprints since then. All family has had time with him in person or talking to him with the phone to his ear. We in the family are well, too, although weary in the waiting, but **much is happening in the lives of those who love Dale** through expressing love, sorrow, and forgiveness. We are thankful for those who need/want time to talk with him and us.

> **NOTE: On Sunday, Lin asked if I had made arrangements for Dale's request to have his body donated for**

medical research. I had not and did not know the process. What I did know is that in grad school at the University of Florida, Dale had reason and opportunity to work in that lab area as he pursued a minor in Anatomy and Physiology. Those lab sessions he found most valuable and determined early on that he would donate his body to that end. I honor that and trust God to oversee the outworking in every way.

Monday, I intended to pursue the process and was immediately assisted by a hospice social worker who asked what help she could be for me. I told her that I only knew that UF was the place to start, and she took it from there. By late afternoon, I had the information needed and the paperwork was being sent.

Tuesday, I spent most of the day in the grueling process of reading and filling out the paperwork, much of which brought things to mind that were difficult to deal with emotionally. The hospice staff was WONDERFUL in assisting me in every possible way with office needs, food, hugs, compassion, a notary, and faxing the paperwork. By the end of the day, Dale's wishes were completed, and I was drained. *I was grateful to be able to tell him all was finished.* Then I went home and left him in the care of my sister Nancy and the hospice staff overnight.

8/15/2018 His Forever Home

Dale gave up his earthly life and moved to his new "home" at 5:30 a.m. All was truly finished for him on this earth. In typical Dale fashion, he arose early in the morning. Our teacher daughter and school-age grandkids were still at home. We all gathered at my home for a memorable day together, crying and laughing and including Dale comfortably in the conversations. We are blessed.

...I know not what the future holds, but I know Who holds the future.

8/16/2018 From Christy

Yesterday morning, August 15th, Heaven gained an amazing coach, teacher, and man when my daddy went to be with Jesus. He was my dad, my mentor, my teacher, and my hero. He really seemed like superman to so many around him and it's hard to believe he's gone.

He taught me everything that I know about my profession. I have tried hard to follow in his footsteps as a science teacher and volleyball coach. My heart has been overwhelmed by all the comments from former players and students about Coach Hutch. It has truly inspired me, and I pray that I can have even a fraction of the impact that he had during his life.

My dad was also the most generous person that I have ever known. He would do anything for anybody. Since both my parents were teachers, we grew up with very little money but that didn't stop my dad. He never said no to a person who was truly in need. We had people move in with us, gave a family a vehicle, left clothing on the doorstep for people in need...the examples are endless.

Epilogue

August 15, 2019 - One Year Later (Last Caring Bridge Entry)

When I awoke this Thursday, it was storming outside and there was thunder, lightning, and rain on the metal roof. It was fitting for a time of reflection, but I had plans to be out on David's boat today. Once again, I yielded to God's timing, even welcomed it. If I've learned anything over the past five years, it's to wait on God for the next step, without grumbling. He certainly knows better than I do. I had spent the night here at David's, so I sat on the front porch with the patter of rain and call of the birds, thankful for a break in the heat and touched by the breeze. Dale and I built this house in 1989; now David and Stephanie have lived here longer than we did! But it's still one of my favorite places in a storm, especially the front porch.

So, I'm reflecting on this first year with Dale being gone. After forty-nine plus years of being together, Dale is evident in the very fabric of my life and is comfortably present in many conversations with family and friends. He's there in the expressions and gestures of his kids and grandkids. His stories and jokes are repeated to us by friends and students as well as among family. "Dale-isms" coming from loved ones make us chuckle (and sometimes snicker). His favorites such as good music (with great sound, of course), Gator football, Gulf Coast HS volleyball, Star Wars, Star Trek, ice cream, fishing and fresh fish, health and nutrition, and anything relating to science, coastal living and Florida history serve as colorful pieces of the Hutcherson tapestry and continue to weave their way into our days and months.

From the porch, I spotted a wading bird in the ditch below, happy with what he's been given this morning. I'm happy, too, with what God provides for me; my life this year has been full, more than I'd ever imagined... and I am well.

THANKFUL - that last August when our family realized that we could no longer have peace and safety for Dale at home, that God carried him, and us and the Steens for two weeks through the process of taking Dale to the Home He had prepared for him. THANKFUL.

RESTORED - from the emotional upheaval, physical strain, and social drought of four years of caregiving. All in good time, God's time. Grieving has been processing for five years now and takes many forms. I may be fragile, but not weak; alone, but not lonely; undecided, but not confused. I've regained physical strength, stabilizing muscles and endurance; normalized in social conversation; become accustomed to travel and driving long distances once again. These things have long been a part of my life but had been hidden away as our life became more confined to house and neighborhood. After these past few years of enjoying music and movies familiar to Dale for his comfort, I am now happily listening to new music/artists and catching up with movies and documentaries of the past few years. At Christmas, I confronted and gratefully overcame tentative feelings about singing in public again without the lifelong benefit of Dale's encouragement and critique. Restoration of my emotional health even allowed me to sing *"My Heart Will Go On"* from Titanic for the spring chorus program. Although I experience an array of emotions, God's shalom/peace reigns in my heart. He offers safety, rest, prosperity, wholeness, welfare, completion, fullness, soundness, and well-being. RESTORED. How can I not be grateful?

AMAZED - at the plans God has unfolded for me. "Oh, the places you'll go!" Visits and travels, leaf-peeping, camping, sisters' visit in the snow, Garth Brooks at the Swamp, ISRAEL, Baltic cruise, Colorado, Mercy Me at Red Rocks Amphitheater, and Philadelphia. AMAZING places, sights, and insights beyond what I could imagine!

"From the highest of heights to the depths of the sea, Creation's revealing Your majesty"

(Indescribable by Chris Tomlin)[5]

Within six weeks:
- I visited the Dead Sea, *lowest land elevation on earth at 1,412 ft below sea level...*
- AND THEN visited Leadville, CO, which, at an *elevation of 10,152 ft above sea level, has the highest elevation of any incorporated US city.*

Me...whose home is Englewood at just 10 ft above sea level!! AMAZED.

BLESSED - by Dale's provision of a safe and social residential community in which I can heal as well as help. The comfort of living in Englewood with roots that go deep and relationships I can trust. The privilege of living near our son David's family and enjoying three grandsons' activities and personal growth. The advantage of being well-suited to road trips (thanks, Mom and Dad), allowing me to be a part of our daughter Christy's "volleyball family" ninety minutes down the road. The blessing of our oldest grandson Joshua entering college this week at UF in Gainesville, following his Papa's footsteps and giving me opportunity to reconnect with the town and friends that I hold so dear. Renewed friendships, conversations with Dale's Gator football teammates, my 50th class reunion, orchid

---

[5] (Tomlin 2004)

show with my college roommate, Christmas caroling with Aphasia Support friends, a weekend with college dormmates, Solo Sisters' lunches, reconnecting in Copenhagen with Mette, our Danish foreign exchange student from the 80s. What rich relationships! I am BLESSED.

CHANGED - Yes, change is a familiar friend. Dale and I both changed much as we grew together, and that continues. I find myself more patient, a better listener, and bold in the face of fear (thank the Lord). I rely on others more quickly to help me as needed, even in personal areas. Dale is no longer here to give his insight/opinion, so I turn to family and friends. My conversational habits had changed as I needed to speak for Dale when he couldn't; consequently, this had caused me to finish others' sentences as well... or to interrupt...which is not a pretty revelation, especially for a former teacher of communication for many years! Working on changing that... reminders are welcome, truly. As for activities, I've taken up square dancing, learned to use a Concept 2 rower/erg for exercise, made new friends in Germany, and delighted in opportunities to be spontaneous! CHANGED.

AVAILABLE - We hear much about "giving back," yet individually we have to take the steps to actually make it happen. I am thankful that Dale and I shared the same vision of an open home and open heart, ready for God to use as He desires, Dale leading the way through his outstanding generosity and me following my parents' example of welcoming others to share whatever we have. In continuing to live out that vision this year, I had the privilege of caring for my dear soul sister after surgery, and for my brother-in-law Bill during his medical procedure as well. Later, my heart and need for affection were filled by helping for a week with my friend's two grandchildren, and more recently for a week with my nephew Dan's four precious children. These opportunities surely served to keep me flexible and from getting stuck in my own ways - a good thing! Although God's days for Dale were finished and he lived them well, God's days for me are NOT finished yet or I wouldn't be here! I remain available for Him to use me as He sees fit, whether as a spouse of forty-seven years, nurturing my children and then grandchildren and any others God brought my way, decades of teaching/working, four years of quite confined caregiving, and now working two days a week helping in the office of friends, all the while supporting family however I can. Wherever He leads, I am AVAILABLE.

LOVED - by God Who continues to show His loving care for me when I least expect it by filling my soul with beauty, music, and freedom; I can't thank Him enough. The kindness of helpful neighbors. Driving around old Sarasota neighborhoods and hangouts. Coming across the perfect little electric fireplace. Receiving Christmas gifts of music and travel. Finding my favorite lilacs on a blustery Helsinki day... AND in an out-of-the-way churchyard in CO. The astounding beauty of little European towns. A chance meeting of my family in the center of Berlin!! An excellent St. Petersburg, Russia, folksong/dance production. A boat ride on the Sea of Galilee... and then realizing God made that plan and paved the way for me to be baptized/immersed in that very Sea. It was a new birth, a fresh start exactly nine months after Dale's passing! I could never have caused that to happen; and yet, He cared enough to arrange for me to be in Israel for that experience. LOVED.

I look forward to what He has next for me. Right now Redding, Marceline, Columbus, Phoenix, Oberammergau, and Sackets Harbor are on my "radar."

At this point, I don't expect to journal through Caring Bridge any longer. It has been a joy for me to have you dear friends support and love me and Dale through Caring Bridge. I pray for you and yours that you know Father's love for you, that God will draw you closer to Him and richly bless your days.

Afterword

Now as this journal is ready for the publication process, I find myself again immersed in those four years, having spent many thoughtful hours revisiting and sometimes reliving the experiences about which I was writing. Once again, I've been changed... by the same events through grieving, having new insight, allowing repressed emotions to be dealt with as they surfaced, carefully considering what to share and how others could be helped by our story. From the first thought of writing and sharing publicly the trials and successes of those years, helping others has always been foremost in my mind. There is no other reason to share, to emotionally walk through those hard times, except that others might gain encouragement, knowledge, and insight, the very things I needed on October 3, 2014, and the following four years.

As Dale and I built our family with a foundation of openly sharing our lives and our homes with love and transparency, in the post-stroke years I/we continued to openly share with others in need from what we learned, both when Dale was still with us and after he had passed. This will continue; it is who I am, inseparably integrated with who Dale was through the oneness of our forty-seven-year marriage. What happens after publication remains to be seen; presently, I have two other related books in process to offer hope and resources in the midst of a trial, specifically trauma, stroke, TBI, aphasia and dementia. God has seen fit to extend my days on this earth and I will fully live those days to the benefit of families, serving God and others with purpose, broadcasting the weighty knowledge of my life experience, bringing clarity and encouragement, speaking Truth and Life, and choosing Joy.

Donna Hutcherson

January, 2022

Appendix One

RESOURCE LIST

STROKE:
The Brain That Changes Itself: Stories of Personal Triumph from the Frontiers of Brain Science, *Norman Doidge*, 2007
- actual amazing case studies pioneering the work on brain neuroplasticity

The Brain's Way of Healing Itself, *Norman Doidge*, 2015
- remarkable discoveries and recoveries from the frontiers of neuroplasticity

The Ghost in My Brain, *Clark Elliott PhD*, 2015
- how a Concussion Stole My Life and How the New Science of Brain Plasticity Helped Me Get It Back

LEFT neglected, *Lisa Genova*, 2011
- a novel insightfully describing the character's left side neglect due to TBI after a car accident

My Stroke of Insight: A Brain Scientist's Personal Journey, *Jill Bolte Taylor, PhD*, 2006.

Never Give Up: My Stroke, My Recovery, and My Return to the NFL, *Tedy Bruschi*, 2007.

Return to Ithaca: A Woman's Triumph Over the Disabilities of a Severe Stroke, *Barbara Newborn*, 1997

SPARK! Dr. John J. Ratey and Eric Hagerman, 2008
- how exercise will improve the performance of your brain

Switch on Your Brain, *Dr. Caroline Leaf*, 2013

-a communication pathologist and audiologist who has worked in the area of cognitive neuroscience since 1985, including pioneering work on neuroplasticity

True Strength: My Journey from Hercules to Mere Mortal--and How Nearly Dying Saved My Life, *Kevin Sorbo*, 2011.
-memoir of transformation, persistence, and hope after suffering strokes at age thirty-eight

RELATED RESOURCES:

After This..., *Marcus Engel*, 2006,
-recovery after severe injury and blindness from an auto accident

Beautiful Battlefields, *Bo Stern*, 2013 -story of her husband's battle with ALS

Healing Back Pain: The Mind-Body Connection, *John E. Sarno*, 1992

The Healing Brain, *Robert Ornstein PhD and David Sobel MD*, 1987

I'm Here: Compassionate Communication in Patient Care, *Marcus Engel*, 2010

Living with Stroke: A Guide for Families, *Richard C. Senelick MD*, 2010

Sitting Kills, Moving Heals: How Everyday Movement Will Prevent Pain, Illness, and Early Death - and Exercise Alone Won't, *Joan Vernikos,* 2011
-cites her original NASA research on how weightlessness weakens astronauts' muscles, bones, and overall health

Stronger, *Jeff Bauman*, 2014 -the Boston Marathon bomb went off at his feet

Teepa Snow, https://teepasnow.com
- Teepa's life mission is to shed a positive light on dementia. Her Positive Approach to Care® offers help to enhance life and relationships of those living with brain change by

fostering an inclusive global community. Many of her videos are on YouTube.

PHYSICAL HELPS:
Bal-A-Vis-X, *Bill Hubert,* www.bal-a-vis-x.com
    -rhythmic Balance/Auditory/Vision eXercises for brain and brain/body integration
Brain Gym, www.braingym.org
    -educational kinesiology; dedicated to enhancing living and learning through the science of movement.
Dr. Deborah Zelinsky – mindeye.com
Dr. Donalee Markus – designsforstrongminds.com
NeuroAcoustic.com - produces and educates on using sound for stress reduction, relaxation, sleep enhancement, mega-learning, creativity and more.
Never Leave the Playground, *Stephen Jepsen,* www.neverleavetheplayground.com
    -activities (videos) that stimulates the growth of the brain and body by specific training of the hands and feet to promote good health and to have fun

Appendix Two

DEFINITION OF TERMS

AFib	Atrial Fibrillation, a type of arrhythmia or abnormal heartbeat
Bal-A-Vis-X	Balance/Auditory/Vision eXercises, all deeply rooted in rhythm
BP	Blood Pressure
Caring Bridge	a personal health journal website
CT or CAT scan	diagnostic medical imaging test using X-rays and a computer
CNA	Certified Nursing Assistant
CRU	Comprehensive Rehab Unit
DMV	Department of Motor Vehicles
EEG	Electroencephalogram - test to evaluate the brain's electrical activity
ECG/EKG	Electrocardiogram test that measures the heart's electrical activity
EMS/EMT	Emergency Medical Services/ Technician
ESE	Exceptional Student Education, specially designed instruction and related services for children with disabilities
FGCU	Florida Gulf Coast University - state university in Estero, FL
FSU	Florida State University - state university in Tallahassee, FL
GCHS	Gulf Coast High School - in Naples, FL

HBOT	Hyperbaric Oxygen Therapy
HH	Homonymous Hemianopsia - visual field deficits in same halves of each eye
ICU	Intensive Care Unit
IV	Intravenous - administering medicines or fluids by injecting into a vein
MM	Medical Marijuana
MOSI	Museum of Science and Industry
NPO	taking nothing by mouth
NSF	NeuroRehab Service of Florida
OT	Occupational Therapy
PA	Physician Assistant
PPG	PPG, Inc. in Pittsburgh, PA
PRN	taken as needed, as in medication
PF	Park Forest, residential neighborhood
REM	Rapid Eye Movement, a stage of sleep important for learning and memory
SICU	Stroke Intensive Care Unit
SLP	Speech-Language Pathologist
SMH	Sarasota Memorial Hospital
TBI	Traumatic Brain Injury; stroke is an Acquired Brain Injury (ABI)
TEE	Transesophageal echocardiography -test that produces pictures of the heart using high-frequency sound waves
TLC	Tender, loving care
tPA	tissue plasminogen activator, known as a "clot-buster" drug
UF	University of Florida - state university in Gainesville, FL
USF	University of South Florida - state university in Tampa, FL
UT	University of Tampa -private university in Tampa, FL

Bibliography

American Dictionary of the English Language. n.d. *Definition of consider.* Accessed February 2022. http://www.webstersdictionary1828.com/Dictionary/consider.

Cowman, L.B. 31. *Streams in the Desert.* December 1999. Accessed February 2022. https://www.youdevotion.com/streams/december/31.

—. 1999. *Streams in the Desert.* June 15. Accessed February 2022. https://www.youdevotion.com/streams/june/15.

Taylor, Jill Bolte. 2006. "My Stroke of Insight ." 75. New York, New York: Penquin Books.

Taylor, Jill Bolte. 2006. "My Stroke of Insight." 75. New York, New York: Penguin Books.

Taylor, Jill Bolte. 2006. "My Stroke of Insight." Appendix b. New York, New York: Penguin Books.

The Aphasia Center. n.d. *What's the difference between Aphasia and Apraxia? .* Accessed February 2022. https://theaphasiacenter.com/2019/09/aphasia-and-apraxia/.

Tomlin, Chris. 2004. *Indescribable.* Comp. Laura Story.

About the Author

Donna Hutcherson is a wife, mother, grandmother, and a child of God. She graduated from the University of Florida and taught high school English for 14 years before transitioning to a business career with Walsworth Publishing. She and Dale, her husband of 47 years, raised their two children in southwest Florida and openly shared their home to meet the needs of many. In the local church, Donna served in many capacities including worship leader and Bible teacher and is a graduate of Gospel Crusade's Institute of Ministry and a student at online School of Kingdom.

Through the Fire is her first book in a series for caregivers.

Website   for-those-who-care.com

Facebook   facebook.com/groups/990074124956976

Website

Facebook